THE
Outward Bound®
WILDERNESS
FIRST-AID
HANDBOOK

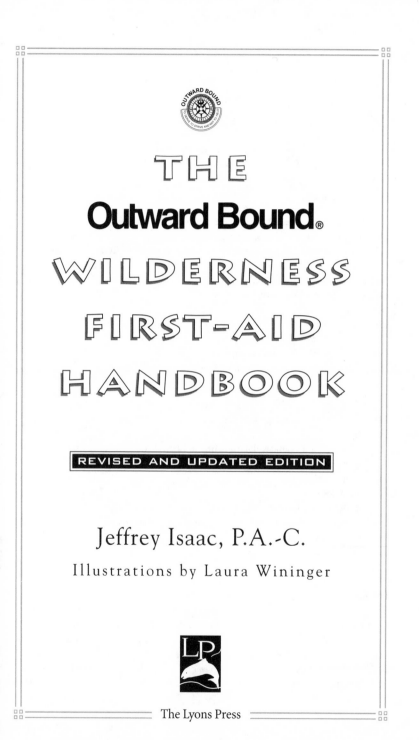

THE
Outward Bound®
WILDERNESS
FIRST-AID
HANDBOOK

REVISED AND UPDATED EDITION

Jeffrey Isaac, P.A.-C.

Illustrations by Laura Wininger

The Lyons Press

To those in the field

Copyright © 1998 by Jeffrey Isaac and Peter Goth
Illustrations copyright © 1998 by Laura Wininger
All Rights Reserved. No part of this book may be reproduced in any manner without the express written consent of the publisher, except in the case of brief excerpts in critical reviews and articles. All inquiries should be addressed to: The Lyons Press, 31 West 21 Street, New York, New York 10010.

Outward Bound® is a registered trademark of Outward Bound, Inc.

Printed in the United States of America
Design and composition by Rohani Design, Edmonds, Washington

10 9 8 7 6 5 4 3 2

Library of Congress Cataloging-in-Publication Data
Isaac, Jeff.
     The outward bound wilderness first-aid handbook / by Jeffrey Isaac; illustra-
tions by Laura Wininger.—Rev. and updated ed.
       p. cm.
     Includes index.
     ISBN 1-55821-682-0 (pb)
     1. First aid in illness and injury—Handbooks, manuals, etc. 2. Outdoor med-
ical emergencies—Handbooks, manuals, etc. I. Title. RC88.9.095I82 1998
     616.02'52—dc21   97-43329
                                                                        CIP

Publisher's Note
The information contained in this book is intended to serve as a guide for those who may need to provide first aid. It is not intended to be a substitute for professional medical advice or training. The authors disclaim any responsibility or liability for any loss that may occur as a result of information, procedures, or techniques included in this work. *Few would venture into the woods not knowing how to pitch a tent or light a stove—first-aid training is equally essential knowledge and should be an integral part of all trip planning.*

CONTENTS

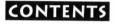

PREFACE

Wilderness medicine is a field full of impressive characters. At any conference, you will find yourself surrounded by people who have climbed Everest, run field hospitals in Somalia, and generally pushed the limits of adventure and medicine all over the planet. There are experts in high-altitude medicine, dive medicine, tropical diseases, and combat medicine. There are people who are prolific authors, and work the lecture circuit, and people who practice quietly in the uncivilized corners of the globe.

My favorite character of them all is Peter Goth, an emergency physician with his own list of impressive accomplishments and publications. But it is not the list that has earned my admiration, it is his ability to explain the workings of the human body, and the principles of emergency medical care, in a commonsense, practical way that anyone can appreciate and understand. This gift, coupled with his belief that medical knowledge belongs to everyone, made him an inspiring teacher and well-respected spokesman in the emerging field of wilderness medicine.

In the early 1980s, Dr. Goth led the design and development of a wilderness-medicine program for Outward Bound instructors. The first courses were taught at the Hurricane Island School, but quickly became the standard of training throughout the Outward Bound system in the United States. During this period, Dr. Goth founded Wilderness Medical Associates, Inc., a company that has grown to become one of the largest wilderness-medicine training organizations in the world.

All of this happened, I believe, because his teaching philosophy appeals to such a wide range of individuals, from experienced physicians to laypeople with no medical training at all. Its focus is on helping the student understand the principles of body function in health and in injury, and how this general knowledge can be applied to a wide variety of medical problems. The backcountry setting of these courses served to accentuate the elemental nature of medicine, and to stimulate the desire to understand it. The first edition of this book was based on the course curriculum developed during this first decade of teaching experience, and was a joy to produce.

In the years since its publication, interest in wilderness medicine has continued to grow rapidly. New committees have formed, new protocols and certifications have sprouted like weeds, and the companies and individuals offering training now number in the hundreds. Experts are everywhere, and there is no shortage of opinions about things that should be done. In this environment, the revised and updated edition was far more difficult to write.

In spite of some changes in terminology, however, I am pleased to say that the original style remains, and has even been improved. The book continues to stress the understanding of principles over the memorization of protocols, and the triumph of common sense over dogma. I am hopeful, maybe even confident, that the subject of wilderness medicine, and the way it is presented here, will continue to enjoy wide acceptance.

WHY THE
OUTWARD BOUND®
WILDERNESS FIRST-AID HANDBOOK

Hikers, backpackers, campers, fishermen, canoe trippers, climbers, and anyone who ventures into the wilderness areas of our country can benefit from the information in this practical book.

Since 1961, Outward Bound USA has been running courses for young people and adults in spectacular wilderness and backcountry areas. Over 450,000 people have graduated from Outward Bound programs—now more than 30,000 annually. The safety of students and staff is of utmost concern and is our most important priority.

With well-qualified staff leading tens of thousands of novice outdoorspeople in a variety of wilderness activities in the back-country, we have had to cope with a wide variety of emergencies both with our students as well as during our traditional search-and-rescue missions.

This book has been developed in conjunction with professionals such as Wilderness Medical Associates as a practical and useful guide to all those enthusiasts who use our country's wilderness areas. When you can't call 911 to ask for Emergency Medical Services to come to your assistance, the information in this book will increase your competence and confidence in dealing with an emergency.

It is Outward Bound's hope that with the knowledge available in this book, you who travel in remote areas will be able to react more confidently in emergency situations, thereby enhancing the enjoyment and personal renewal found in wilderness activities.

Lewis R. Glenn
Vice President of Safety and Program
Outward Bound USA

ABOUT
OUTWARD BOUND®

Outward Bound is the largest and oldest adventure-based educational institution in the world and is a nonprofit, tax-exempt organization. Best known for its ability to build participants' self-confidence and self-reliance, Outward Bound also develops a sense of compassion for others, responsibility to the community, sensitivity to the environment, and leadership skills in individuals from many different backgrounds.

Outward Bound uses challenging activities, primarily in wilderness settings, to teach both adults and young people more about themselves and others and to help them realize that many of their preconceived limits are self-imposed.

Each Outward Bound course centers around challenging activities for which extensive technical training is given. Included among more than 700 courses offered to people fourteen years of age and older are experiences ranging in diversity from sailing, backpacking, canoeing, sea kayaking, and white-water rafting to mountain climbing, skiing, dogsledding, and even urban experiences. All use the vast majestic wilderness areas of twenty-two states as well as selected urban environments in major U.S. cities. Traditional Outward

Bound course elements include map and compass use, rock climbing, rappelling, and Leave No Trace camping and traveling techniques.

A BRIEF HISTORY

Outward Bound grew out of the need to instill a spiritual tenacity and the will to survive in young British seamen being torpedoed by German U-boats during World War II. From this beginning in 1941, a number of Outward Bound schools were established in the United Kingdom. The movement soon spread to Europe, Africa, Asia, Australia, and North America. Today there are more than fifty Outward Bound schools and centers on five continents.

The first Outward Bound school in the United States was established in 1961 in Colorado. Now there are five U.S. Outward Bound schools: Colorado; Hurricane Island, in Maine; North Carolina; Pacific Crest, in Oregon; and Voyageur, in Minnesota.

Outward Bound has also established a number of urban programs currently operating in Atlanta, Baltimore, Boston, and New York City. These urban programs have been specifically designed to address the needs of inner-city youth and the social, cultural, and educational problems existing in every large city throughout the country.

SERVING SPECIAL POPULATIONS

A typical Outward Bound course is from four to nine days for adults, and from three to four weeks for high school and college students. Outward Bound also offers courses specifically developed to serve the unique requirements of some special populations: troubled youth and people with special medical needs, for example. At each school, courses incorporating leadership development and wilderness study may be taken for college credit, and there are also specific courses for professional and managerial groups.

SAFETY IN THE WILDERNESS

All Outward Bound instructors are highly skilled and experienced in wilderness adventure. Training includes the latest technical and safety management practices. Outward Bound's enviable safety record reflects the emphasis each school places on ensuring the well-being of students entrusted to its care.

BENEFITS

After an Outward Bound experience, participants discover many positive attributes about themselves. All expect more from themselves. They become confident whereas before they were hesitant. They learn to share, to lead and to follow, and to work together as a group. In safeguarding one another, they form bonds of mutual trust. They discover that many problems can be solved only with the cooperation of all members of a group.

Over the past half-century, research has validated these universally recognized positive effects on personal growth. Outward Bound is well known for its ability to enhance confidence and interpersonal relationships, develop leadership skills, and has been shown to provide marked improvements in many other ares of personal and moral development, such as self-esteem, assertiveness, and dependability.

As one Outward Bound student said: "We are better than we know. If we can be made to see it, perhaps for the rest of our lives we will be unwilling to settle for less."

For further information please call, write, or E-mail Outward Bound USA, Route 9D, R2 Box 280, Garrison, NY 10524, toll-free (800) 243-8520, E-mail: national@outwardbound.org. Visit the Outward Bound USA Web site at: http://www.outwardbound.org.

INTRODUCTION

The expedition is over and my students are returning to life ashore—some reluctantly, some delighted to be back. I'm looking forward to spending some time on my own. Teaching an Outward Bound course is an exercise in perpetual responsibility that I accept gladly but surrender with equal enthusiasm when it is finished. I now have an appointment with fourteen miles of up-country white water.

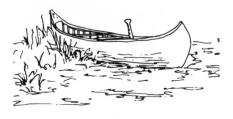

The back of my pickup is packed with wet suits, gloves, piles of polypropylene, and the rest of the paraphernalia associated with spring paddling in Maine. Crowning the heap is my battered canoe. Her scars are a cumulative history of all of the rocks, stumps, and other boats we've encountered over the years. In reality she is damaged equipment. But in spirit she is a symbol of both the joys and miseries of my encounters with the river.

My own bumps, bruises, and wounds have healed. Fortunately, all were minor. If they weren't, I hope that I'd view them with the same degree of respect and acceptance. Risk is part of the game, and injury is one of the consequences.

This weekend thousands of paddlers, climbers, and hikers will head out looking for excitement, relaxation, and adventure. And though some of them will suffer mishaps, the perceived risks in such activities are usually much greater than the actual danger. This is certainly true in the carefully controlled environment of an Outward Bound Program.

Nevertheless, we all understand that in many worthwhile activities there are real dangers. In Outward Bound courses, we strive to balance these dangers against the joys and benefits of intimate experience with wild country and natural forces. This is the sensitive balance known as "acceptable risk." Hazards are not sought for their own sake, but neither are they completely avoided. For backcountry travelers, a critical part of striking the balance is the ability to handle dangerous situations when they occur. This includes a logical, commonsense approach to injury and illness that takes into account the unique aspects of the wilderness setting.

In our "civilized" settings we delegate this responsibility to trained professionals. It is the business of paramedics, nurses, physician assistants, and medical doctors to recognize medical emergencies and know what to do about them. This system allows everyone else to get by with knowing very little and yet still keep the risk of daily living within the range of "acceptable." But once one leaves the civilized world behind, the situation changes dramatically. Techniques and equipment developed for the emergency room or ambulance are often inappropriate or unavailable outside the hospital. In many wilderness scenarios a team of sled dogs would be more useful than a team of surgeons.

Getting an injured person in the wilderness out to civilized medical care is rarely easy. Even when it's performed by skilled rescuers, a backcountry evacuation is difficult, expensive, and often hazardous. Contrary to the common television image of helicopters swooping to the rescue, such operations are the exception, not the rule. Instead, the "heroic" rescue is usually an arduous, sweaty, muddy scramble that disrupts the lives of dozens of people.

The object in preparing for backcountry medical problems is not to find more and better ways to yell for help, nor is it to stuff your pack with specialty first-aid kits. It is to develop a good basic understanding of the body's structure and functions and to learn some basic techniques for preserving them in the presence of injury.

It is, of course, important to recognize that there are considerable limits to your ability to affect the outcome of some medical emergencies. There are times when screaming for help is absolutely the right thing to do, and times when all the help in the world won't make any difference. The vast majority of situations, however, are well within the capabilities of every backcountry traveler to handle. It is your right and responsibility to know, at least in general terms, how your body works and how to fix it when it's broken.

Like all things remote from civilization, wilderness medicine is elemental. The most important skill is improvisation, and good improvisation requires a solid understanding of the principles behind the treatment. It's a skill like reading a river, or steering a boat in a breaking sea—the technical information is important, but it's the gut feeling for the undertaking that gets you through. This book is designed to introduce the important principles as well as to share the gut feelings of a lot of experienced people. It represents the collective wisdom of literally hundreds of medical practitioners, outdoor educators, sailors, and wilderness travelers. It is offered to you not just as a reference but as part of a lifelong process of learning. We hope that *The Outward Bound Wilderness First-Aid Handbook* will inspire you to further your own medical education and competence. You are, after all is said and written, your own responsibility.

SECTION I

The Approach

to Wilderness

Medical Problems

1

GENERAL PRINCIPLES
IN WILDERNESS MEDICINE

Practical preparation for medical emergencies requires a sound comprehension of the principles behind the procedures. Once you have accomplished this you will never forget what to do because you will *understand* what needs to be done. These principles are mostly common sense and basic knowledge and will turn up again and again to guide you through your study and practice of wilderness emergency care.

Principle: Three Major Body Systems. The organs of the circulatory, respiratory, and nervous systems perform the vital functions that are most essential to life. These systems are interdependent, like the legs of a three-legged stool—you can't survive without all three working together.

Problems with one major body system are quickly reflected in the other two. For example, a serious respiratory system problem, such as an asthma attack, will not only bring about the expected respiratory distress, but it will also produce an increased heart rate (circulatory system) and changes in consciousness (nervous system). Any injury or illness that threatens the vital functions of a major body system is a threat to life. *A major problem with a major body system is a major emergency.*

Principle: Oxygenation and Perfusion. It is the task of the respiratory system to supply outside air to the alveoli of the lungs, where oxygen can enter the blood stream, "filling up" the red blood cells. Adequate oxygenation requires adequate respiration.

The circulatory system transports blood to and from all parts of the body. Blood is carried away from the heart to the smallest blood vessels, called capillaries, where it is forced into the body tissue. This is called "perfusion," and it allows an exchange to take place between the blood and cells—blood gives up oxygen and nutrients to the cells and receives carbon dioxide, water, and wastes to be expelled from the body. Considerable pressure, generated by the pumping action of the heart and constriction of blood vessels, is required to push the blood through the capillary beds. Adequate perfusion requires adequate perfusion pressure.

All living tissue, especially the organs of the major body systems, must be continuously perfused with oxygenated blood. Anything that interferes with this is a real problem. *The preservation of perfusion and oxygenation is the key to successful treatment.*

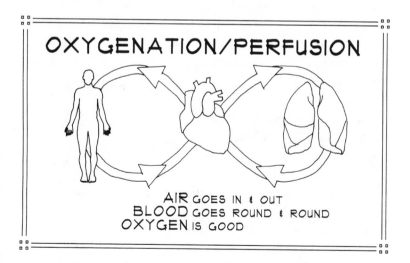

OXYGENATION/PERFUSION

AIR GOES IN & OUT
BLOOD GOES ROUND & ROUND
OXYGEN IS GOOD

Principle: Compensation. The nervous system regulates the function of the circulatory and respiratory systems to maintain adequate perfusion and oxygenation under a variety of conditions.

Heart rate, respiration, and blood vessel constriction are adjusted by the brain to compensate for effects of exercise, environment, injury, and other factors. Adequate compensation requires an intact and functioning nervous system.

The best way to watch compensation in action is to observe vital signs. The basic vital signs are: pulse rate, respiratory rate and effort, level of consciousness and mental status, blood pressure, skin color and warmth, and body core temperature. Minor changes will occur as a healthy body adapts to various stresses of normal life. *Large or persistent changes in vital signs indicate that the body is compensating for abnormal stress, such as injury or illness.*

Principle: Shell/Core Effect. One of the primary compensation mechanisms seen in stress and injury is the shunting of blood from the less-vital organs of the shell to the vital core of the body. This is accomplished by the constriction of the arteries supplying blood to the shell and the dilation of the arteries feeding the core. The shell is composed of the skin, digestive system, and skeletal musculature. The core includes the organs of the major body systems: the brain, heart, lungs, liver, and kidneys.

The shell/core effect accounts for the cool pale skin observed as an early sign of potentially life-threatening volume shock, which is most often caused by a decrease in the volume of circulating blood due to bleeding or dehydration. It can also be the normal and healthy response to a cold environment. In any case, shell/core effect indicates that the body is trying to preserve perfusion of the core organs at the expense of the shell. *Reduced perfusion of the body shell will usually be followed by reduced perfusion of the body core.*

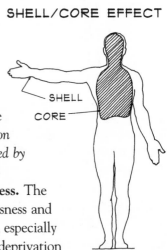

SHELL/CORE EFFECT

SHELL

CORE

Principle: Level of Consciousness. The most revealing vital sign is consciousness and mental status. Nervous system tissue, especially the brain, is very sensitive to oxygen deprivation and will often be first to show the effects of developing problems with perfusion or oxygenation. The severity of the symptoms is closely related to the severity of the problem.

Picture the brain as a sort of onion with increasingly complex layers of function from the inside out. The basic vegetative functions of body regulation, breathing, and consciousness are contained in the deeper, more primitive layers. Higher functions, such as personality, judgment, and problem solving, would be located in the outer layers, because they were added later in evolutionary time.

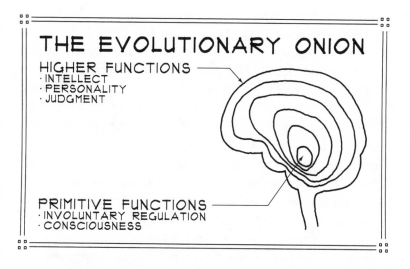

These outer layers, as the most recently acquired, are also the first to be affected when problems develop. The earliest vital-sign changes to be seen are the beginning stages of "peeling the onion." We call this "altered mental status." Patients remain conscious and alert but may become anxious, uncooperative, or respond in ways that don't fit the situation. They may act intoxicated, belligerent, or confused. More extreme injury affects the deeper layers, causing a decrease in level of consciousness. When the onion has peeled this far, the situation has become much more serious. The progression can be reversed if the underlying problems with perfusion and oxygenation are corrected. *Consciousness and mental status are the most reliable indicators of brain perfusion and oxygenation.*

Principle: Ischemia and Infarction. Any body tissue deprived of its oxygen supply will die. Some tissue, like that of the brain, will die within a few minutes. Other tissue, like that of the skin, can last for hours. It seems that the more important an organ is to immediate survival, the more sensitive it is to loss of perfusion and oxygenation.

Ischemia is the term we use for inadequate perfusion: The tissue is not receiving enough oxygen to work properly and survive. Symptoms include pain and impaired function. The chest pain known as angina is caused by ischemia of heart muscle. The facial droop or limb paralysis of a transient ischemic attack (TIA) is caused by ischemia of the part of the brain that controls those muscles. If the ischemia can be quickly reversed or the oxygen demands of the tissue reduced, the pain will go away and function will return.

Prolonged ischemia will inevitably lead to *infarction*, which is the term for tissue death. A heart attack is also called a *myocardial infarction:* the death of heart muscle due to prolonged ischemia. The permanent symptoms of a stroke are due to a cerebral infarction. In limb injuries, prolonged ischemia will also cause tissue infarction and permanent disability. *The symptoms of ischemia are an early warning of serious and permanent problems caused by infarction.*

Principle: Swelling and Pressure. Swelling is caused by the accumulation of excess fluid in body tissues. This can occur almost instantly, in the form of blood escaping from ruptured blood vessels, or slowly, over hours or days, as serum oozes from damaged capillaries as part of the generic inflammatory response to injury or infection (edema). It may be localized, like the swelling of a sprained ankle, or systemic, like the swelling of the whole body that occurs in allergic reactions.

Swelling that develops in a restricted space produces pressure. If the pressure is great enough, it can exceed the perfusion pressure in the circulatory system, preventing the flow of blood. This is exactly what happens to the brain with swelling due to head injury inside the confined space of the skull. It is also responsible for the damage caused by a "compartment syndrome," which can develop inside the muscle compartments of the lower leg after injury. You can create your own compartment syndrome by failing to anticipate the swelling that may develop inside a splint.

Swelling in the confined space of the neck can cause an airway obstruction, preventing oxygen from getting to the lungs. Swelling lower down in the respiratory system can cause airway constriction or pulmonary edema, which will prevent oxygenation of the blood. Airway obstruction or ischemia that affects the vital organs of the major body systems is an immediate threat to life. Prolonged ischemia can also kill nerves and muscle in an arm or leg, causing a permanent disability.

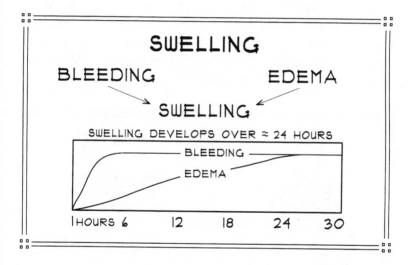

Most of the swelling that occurs following an injury develops during the first six hours, then tapers off over the next eighteen to twenty-four hours. Swelling will increase very little thereafter unless there is a repeat injury or persistent irritation from an infection. *Anticipating and controlling the development of swelling is one of most important aspects of treatment in wilderness medical care.*

Principle: Obstruction and Infection. The human body is full of hollow organs that store, transport, or excrete liquids of all types. These include sweat glands, intestines, bladders, and all of the associated tubing. If the drainage from these organs is obstructed by swelling, deformity, or a foreign body, the fluid buildup and resulting pressure will cause inflammation and pain. If the obstruction lasts long enough, bacteria will begin to grow out of control in the area, and infection will develop. The most common example of this principle is the teenager's worst nightmare, the average pimple, which is an infection of an obstructed sweat gland. Another, more serious, example is appendicitis. *Many serious illnesses have their origins in obstruction.*

Principle: Risk/Benefit Ratio. There is some risk in everything we do. Medical care is no different. Every treatment or decision not to treat, and every emergency evacuation or decision to stay on expedition involves the risk that problems will become worse because of what we've done. Against this risk, we balance the potential benefits of our actions. Good decisions reflect the clear assessment that the potential benefit outweighs the risks to the patient and everyone else involved.

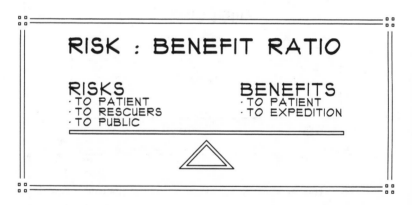

In the backcountry, it is just as important to know when you don't have a medical emergency as when you do. Only a severe problem with a major body system is an extreme emergency. Unfortunately, wilderness and marine rescue is full of stories of high-risk evacuations for low-risk medical problems. Helicopters crash, and rescuers are lost in avalanches while trying to evacuate patients who would have done just fine by waiting a few days. *The ability to objectively weigh this risk/benefit ratio is critical in wilderness medicine.*

Principle: Acute Stress Reaction. A sudden stress or injury that may or may not be serious is often followed by a variety of reactions—including extreme anxiety, disorientation, fainting, hyperventilation, and pain masking—called Acute Stress Reaction (ASR). Sometimes called *psychogenic shock,* ASR is a normal, harmless, and self-limiting nervous system response. The problem with ASR is that it can be mistaken for the symptoms of life-threatening conditions like true shock or head injury or can cause confusion by masking the pain of serious injury. *It is important to be able to distinguish ASR, which is harmless and self-limiting, from true emergencies.*

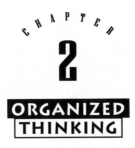

2

ORGANIZED THINKING

Problems, by definition, imply a state of instability. Any problem-solving situation can be improved by the use of an organizational technique that frames the unstable problem within a stable system: in other words, imposing order on chaos.

In the hospital emergency department, clear priorities are established to ensure that the most life-threatening conditions are dealt with immediately by stabilizing and supporting the vital functions of the circulatory, respiratory, and nervous systems. The most significant attention is given to the vitally important and sensitive organs of these major body systems—the heart, lungs, brain, and spinal cord—for they constitute the critical machinery most essential to life. Only after the immediate threats to the patient's life have been stabilized can the process of more specific diagnosis and treatment begin.

The same principle is followed in the backcountry setting. But because in the wilderness we have only basic diagnostic equipment (our hands, eyes, and ears) and limited options for treatment, the medical problems and treatment plans remain basic in nature. This makes things a lot easier from a medical point of view: You don't need to memorize twelve different causes of abdominal pain, you only need to know when to consider abdominal pain potentially serious.

However, unlike the controlled and stable environment of a hospital where the patient's medical problems are the only thing the staff needs to worry about, in the backcountry his or her medical problem is only a small part of a much larger picture that includes weather, terrain, the condition of the other members of the group, available assistance, and a number of other factors. Your treatment plan needs to consider not only medical issues but shelter, transportation, and survival as well.

THE PATIENT ASSESSMENT SYSTEM (PAS)

In the prehospital and backcountry setting, an excellent tool for organized response is the Patient Assessment System (PAS). PAS is based on information gathered in a series of surveys and organized in a standard format. It consists of three important steps: gathering information, organizing a response, and anticipating problems that may develop over time.

SURVEYS—INFORMATION GATHERING

1. Scene Size-up
2. Initial Assessment
3. Focused History and Physical Exam

These are the terms currently in use in the United States Department of Transportation's emergency-medical-technician curriculum to describe the steps taken in our assessment of the scene and the patient. If you have had first-aid training anytime in the past twenty years or so, you will probably recognize these as the Scene Survey, Primary Survey, and Secondary Survey. In other publications and training programs, you may encounter different terms for similar steps in the same process. It doesn't matter what terms you adopt as long as you remember the most important thing—the *concept* of the process.

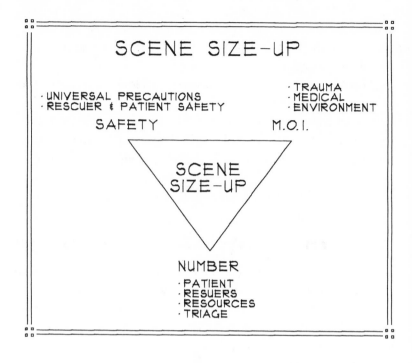

1. SCENE SIZE-UP

RESCUER AND PATIENT SAFETY.

Before rushing to the rescue, be sure you are not going to create more casualties by diving into an unstable situation. You can't help anybody else if you're out of commission yourself. It can take tremendous discipline to overcome the powerful urge to come to the aid of a person in trouble. But this is exactly what you must do—at least for the moment. Stop, look around, and identify all of the hazards. It may be frigid water, another avalanche, or more wasps in the nest. Whatever the situation is, if it can harm you or your fellow rescuers, it must be stabilized before you can do anything else.

In this survey of dangers you must also consider the potential for exposure to blood and other body fluids. A number of diseases can be transmitted this way, including HIV and hepatitis. The use of gloves and eye protection is now standard in all areas of medicine where body-fluid contact is possible. Protecting yourself and others from this kind of exposure is termed "universal precautions."

Once you are safe, or relatively so, look for any further threat to the injured person. Stabilize the scene by moving danger from the patient or the patient from danger. This has priority over everything else that follows. So get him out of the water, out from under the cornice, or away from the wasps before proceeding with evaluation and treatment.

MECHANISM OF INJURY.

Another important element in the survey of the scene is the mechanism of injury. How it happened is usually obvious, but occasionally more investigation will be necessary. For example, how far did she fall? Was it enough of a tumble to cause significant injury? Are there other factors, such as exposure to weather or preexisting illness, that might be the primary reason for the patient's condition?

NUMBER OF PATIENTS.

Determine how many people are injured or at risk. Potentially serious problems are often overlooked in the rush to treat the most noisy and uncomfortable patients. This is especially true in harsh environments, where all the expedition members are at risk for hypothermia or dehydration.

Triage, which is the process of establishing treatment priorities, is important in multiple-casualty situations where resources are limited. This is a good time to avoid "puddle vision": Look beyond that puddle of blood right in front of you and size up the whole scene before deciding where to begin.

2. INITIAL ASSESSMENT

This is your initial quick check on the status of the patient's three major body systems. The critical functions of the circulatory, respiratory, and nervous systems are equally important to survival, and major problems are equally life threatening. The order in which you check and stabilize them will be determined by the situation (not by the order in which they appear on any list).

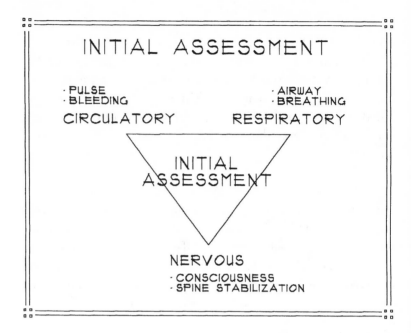

Make sure that the mouth and nose are clear to allow the passage of air and that air is actually going in and out. Be sure that blood is circulating and not running out all over the ground. Also, ensure that the patient's spine is stable, and check the level of consciousness.

Circulatory system:	Check for pulse, look for severe bleeding
Respiratory system:	Clear airway, check for breathing
Nervous system:	Check consciousness, stabilize spine

Performing an Initial Assessment may mean hanging upside down in a crevasse listening for breath sounds in your unconscious partner and looking inside bulky clothing for blood. On the other hand, it may be as simple as asking "How are you doing?" and getting a "Fine" and a smile. Whatever form it takes, it is a critical step in your organized approach to the situation, because any problems encountered in the Initial Assessment must be immediately stabilized before you worry about anything else. You will have to fight the natural tendency to focus on the obvious injuries, like deformed fractures and messy abrasions. This can keep you from finding the life-threatening problems, like airway obstruction or severe bleeding.

The immediate management of life-threatening problems found in the Initial Assessment is referred to as Basic Life Support (BLS) and is covered in Chapter 3. If the situation requires Basic Life Support, you may never be able to go any farther with your patient exam. In most cases, however, you will be able to determine that no life-threatening problem exists and go on to the Focused History and Physical Exam.

3. Focused History and Physical Exam

By now you have decided there is nothing in the current environment that can harm you, the other rescuers, or the injured person and there are no problems in the patient's major body systems that are immediately life threatening. For the moment the scene is stable, and the patient is stable.

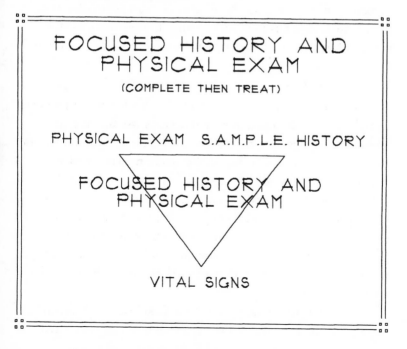

FOCUSED HISTORY AND PHYSICAL EXAM
(COMPLETE THEN TREAT)

PHYSICAL EXAM S.A.M.P.L.E. HISTORY

FOCUSED HISTORY AND PHYSICAL EXAM

VITAL SIGNS

Exam

This stage is a slower, more deliberate examination of the whole patient. It is less urgent than the Initial Assessment, but speed and detail change with circumstances. Unless your Initial Assessment missed something, it is not necessary or efficient to stop and treat problems as you find them. Get the whole picture, complete your list, then return to treat each problem in order of priority.

Although it really makes no difference in what order you do your exam, most people like to start with the head and neck, moving to the chest, abdomen, pelvis, legs, arms, and back. You are looking and feeling for abnormality such as tenderness (pain caused by touch), swelling, deformity, discoloration, or bleeding. You should be gentle, moving the patient as little as possible.

Your exam should be as comprehensive as the situation allows and requires, but common sense should prevail. It is not always necessary to directly see or feel every body part in every patient. If no symptom or mechanism of injury suggests involvement of a particular body part, exposure and examination is not important, especially in the field. What is important is that the rescuer go through a complete head-to-toe checklist, at least in his or her own mind.

Vital Signs

Although the Initial Assessment looks quickly for urgent problems with the circulatory, respiratory, and nervous systems, the vital signs provide more objective measurement of these same three systems over a period of time. Changes in the functioning of the major body systems will be revealed by changes in vital signs, which often follow predictable patterns. You can think of vital signs as the safety net of patient assessment. By measuring the same standard signs at regular intervals, you can get a sense for improvement or decay in a patient's condition. Is your treatment working? Are things getting better or worse? Is it time to panic, or can you sit back and have another handful of gorp?

The detail with which you measure vital signs will depend on the equipment available and your level of training. How often you

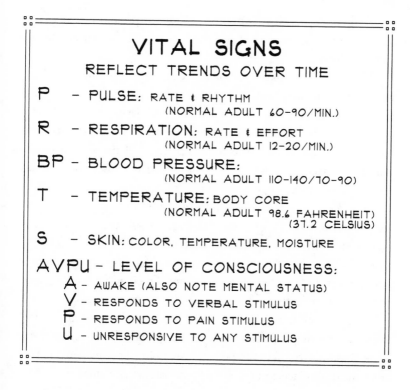

VITAL SIGNS
REFLECT TRENDS OVER TIME

P   – PULSE: RATE & RHYTHM
              (NORMAL ADULT 60-90/MIN.)

R   – RESPIRATION: RATE & EFFORT
              (NORMAL ADULT 12-20/MIN.)

BP – BLOOD PRESSURE:
              (NORMAL ADULT 110-140/70-90)

T   – TEMPERATURE: BODY CORE
              (NORMAL ADULT 98.6 FAHRENHEIT)
                    (37.2 CELSIUS)

S   – SKIN: COLOR, TEMPERATURE, MOISTURE

AVPU – LEVEL OF CONSCIOUSNESS:
    A – AWAKE (ALSO NOTE MENTAL STATUS)
    V – RESPONDS TO VERBAL STIMULUS
    P – RESPONDS TO PAIN STIMULUS
    U – UNRESPONSIVE TO ANY STIMULUS

measure vital signs will depend on the logistical situation and your level of comfort with the patient's condition. Vital signs are listed above, with the range of normal values in parentheses.

Pulse is a very helpful and reliable vital sign; it is easy to measure accurately and reflects almost any change in the circulatory system. Pulse rate is expressed in beats per minute and can be quickly obtained by counting the pulse for fifteen seconds and multiplying that figure by four. Noting the rhythm (irregular or regular) can be helpful in some cases, but subjective comments like "weak," "thready," or "bounding" are rarely useful. You can find the pulse in any artery, but the radial (wrist), carotid (neck), and temporal (temple) arteries are the most commonly used.

Respiratory rate is a direct measurement of respiratory system function, but it can be difficult to measure accurately if the patient is talking or crying. It is expressed in breaths per minute. It is also useful to note the degree of respiratory effort if the patient seems to be in distress.

Blood pressure, like pulse, is an accurate measurement of how well the circulatory system is functioning. A reading of 130/80 would be normal for an adult. The first number (*systolic*) indicates the pressure produced by the force of each heart contraction. The second (*diastolic*) reflects the resting pressure of the system maintained by arterial muscle tone. For emergency use, the systolic pressure is the most important.

Blood pressure is measured by inflating a blood pressure cuff around an arm (or leg) and applying enough pressure to completely stop arterial blood flow. The cuff is then slowly deflated while the examiner watches the gauge and feels for the return of a pulse, or listens for it with a stethoscope. The reading on the gauge when the first beat is felt or heard is the systolic measurement.

Temperature in vital signs refers to the temperature of the vital organs of the major body systems (core temperature). This can be quite different from skin temperature, even in a healthy person. The most accurate place to measure core temperature is in the rectum. Oral temperatures are affected by eating, breathing, and talking and are usually about a degree lower than core temperature.

Skin color and temperature accurately reflects the perfusion of the body shell. It is described according to color, temperature, and moisture. Skin perfusion is reduced whenever vital organ perfusion is reduced. However, keep in mind that cool and pale skin can also be part of a normal response to cold weather.

Consciousness and mental status is a measure of nervous system (brain) function. No special instruments are required to measure it. Consciousness is described as relating to one of four letters on the AVPU scale:

A: Awake

V: Responsive to Verbal stimulus

P: Responsive only to Painful stimulus

U: Unresponsive to any stimulus

This is a widely used and relatively precise description that avoids confusing terms such as "semiconscious" and "in and out."

You can fine-tune your description of awake patients by describing their mental status. This refers to the patient's level of orientation and anxiety. Problems in the nervous system almost always cause some change in mental status well before changes in consciousness. People with normal mental status generally know who they are, where they are, what day it is, and why they are where they are. You'll have to allow some slack for time at sea, of course. We've had perfectly healthy Outward Bound students on long ocean expeditions who are unable to keep track of the month, never mind the day of the week.

When measuring vital signs, it is most important to take all six together at regular intervals and to record the time they were taken. Remember, the value of this assessment safety net is in observing change over time. Even if you don't carry blood pressure cuffs, clinical thermometers, or even a watch, a valuable assessment of vital signs can still be made through relative measurements. For example, pulse can be read as "fast" or "slow," temperature as "cool" or "warm." Blood pressure can be assessed as "normal" or "low" based on signs of adequate or inadequate perfusion (more on this later).

HISTORY

The final act in the process of gathering information is to obtain a relevant history. The mnemonic acronym for the list of questions to ask is SAMPLE:

S: **Symptoms** associated with present problem

A: **Allergies** to insect stings, foods, medications, other

M: **Medication** that the patient is currently taking

P: **Past history** of similar or related problems

L: **Last food and fluids**, time and amounts

E: **Events** leading up to the incident

Performing a comprehensive Focused History and Physical Exam can take some time and may not always be necessary or appropriate. A simple finger laceration doesn't warrant a full-body examination or a discussion of the patient's gallbladder surgery fifteen years ago. However, many accident scenarios are unwitnessed, confused by pain and anxiety, and involve hidden injuries. In these situations, your own level of anxiety as a rescuer may require that you have a familiar structure to function within. This will do a lot to put your mind at ease and stabilize an uncomfortable situation.

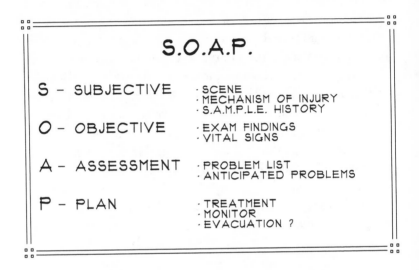

ORGANIZING YOUR RESPONSE—SOAP

The system of organization commonly used by the medical profession is the SOAP format. SOAP is the acronym for Subjective, Objective, Assessment, and Plan. It is a simple and effective management process progressing from the gathering of information through the identification of the problems to the formation of a plan to deal with each problem. This is the way medical records are written and the order in which medical information is communicated. The general meaning of each stage is as follows:

S: **Subjective.** Description of the scene, the mechanism of injury, symptoms the patient is complaining about, relevant history (SAMPLE).

O: **Objective.** What you see, hear, feel, and smell during your examination of the patient. Includes vital signs.

A: **Assessment.** The "problem list" based on the subjective and objective findings.

P: **Plan.** What are you going to do about each problem now? Includes plans for treatments, monitoring the patient's condition, and evacuation, if necessary.

Using this system, a typical brief SOAP for an emergency-room case might look like this:

S: A nine-year-old boy fell off his bicycle when he rode over a curb at slow speed. He complains of pain in his right wrist and tingling in his fingers. He has no complaints of pain anywhere else. No allergies, no medications, no past history of wrist injury, last meal 12:00, fell because he didn't see the curb.

O: An alert, oriented, but uncomfortable boy. The right wrist is swollen and tender to touch. There is no other obvious injury. The patient refuses to move the wrist voluntarily. The fingers are warm and pink and can be wiggled with slight pain felt at the wrist. The patient can feel the light touch of a cotton swab on the end of each finger. X ray shows a buckle fracture of the distal radius (minor break in the end of one of the bones in the forearm).

A: Fracture right wrist.

P: Splint wrist. Follow-up with an orthopedic surgeon in three days. Return to the hospital if fingers become blue or cold or the tingling becomes at all worse.

This format paints a nice picture of the situation. In just a few words you get a sense for who the patient is and what happened, and what the practitioner is going to do about it. There is also a brief description of problems that might occur and what the response should be.

The SOAP format is perfectly adaptable to the backcountry setting, and it performs the same vital function that it does in the emergency room. It organizes your thoughts, imposes order on chaos, and allows you to communicate your ideas and plans to the patient and whoever might be taking care of the patient next.

Anticipated Problems (A')

In the wilderness setting, we need to expand SOAP a little to take into account the unique environment in which we are traveling. We must consider problems created by weather, terrain, distance, and time, all factors just as important to our planning as the condition of the patient. In long-term care, we add a list of *anticipated problems* (A'), which could be complications of the injury itself or the result of exposure to environmental factors. By including A' in the SOAP note we are more likely to prevent problems from developing, or to be ready to deal with them when they can't be avoided.

WATCHING FOR CHANGE—MONITOR

As your patient's condition, the weather, and your logistical situation change with time, plans will need to be revised and communication updated. You will want to repeat the relevant parts of your surveys and revise your SOAP at regular intervals. This is where you watch for the anticipated problems (A') you've listed in your original SOAP note.

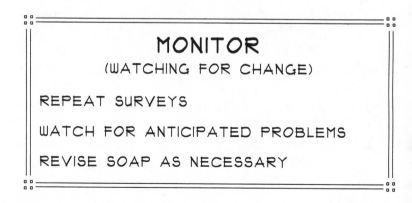

MONITOR
(WATCHING FOR CHANGE)

REPEAT SURVEYS

WATCH FOR ANTICIPATED PROBLEMS

REVISE SOAP AS NECESSARY

Patients with potential major body system problems should be reevaluated most often, at least every fifteen minutes if possible. The status of injured extremities can be checked less frequently, at one- to two-hour intervals. Conditions that develop slowly, such as wound infection, might be adequately monitored every six hours.

Now, with these specialized additions to SOAP in mind, let's take that previous emergency room case into the backcountry:

S: A nine-year-old boy fell onto his outstretched right arm while gathering firewood near the Speck Pond Shelter about one hour ago. He complains of pain in his right wrist and tingling in his fingers. He has no complaints of pain anywhere else. No allergies, no medications, no past history of wrist injury, last meal 12:00. The fall was due to slipping on wet leaves, and not from a significant height. He does not feel cold or hungry. It is now sunset. The air temperature is 60 degrees. It is raining lightly.

O: At 18:30: An alert, responsive, but uncomfortable boy is found sitting on a rock holding his right arm. He is warm, dry, and adequately dressed. His right wrist is slightly swollen and tender to touch, and he is unable to move it. He can wiggle his fingers and feel the light touch of the examiner's hand. His skin color is normal. There is no other obvious injury.

A: Unstable injury right wrist

A': 1. Increased swelling, pressure, ischemia

2. Hypothermia

P: Splint the wrist, keep the patient quiet and the arm elevated.

1. Monitor left hand every two hours, adjust the splint if necessary.

2. Stay in shelter tonight, keep the patient dry and well fed, walk out in daylight tomorrow.

In this example, the anticipated problem of hypothermia is included because it often occurs in wet and cool weather, especially

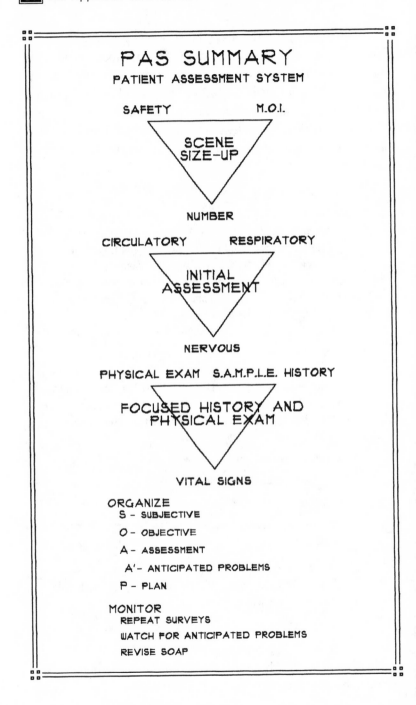

PAS SUMMARY
PATIENT ASSESSMENT SYSTEM

SAFETY   M.O.I.

SCENE SIZE-UP

NUMBER

CIRCULATORY   RESPIRATORY

INITIAL ASSESSMENT

NERVOUS

PHYSICAL EXAM   S.A.M.P.L.E. HISTORY

FOCUSED HISTORY AND PHYSICAL EXAM

VITAL SIGNS

ORGANIZE
  S – SUBJECTIVE
  O – OBJECTIVE
  A – ASSESSMENT
   A' – ANTICIPATED PROBLEMS
  P – PLAN

MONITOR
  REPEAT SURVEYS
  WATCH FOR ANTICIPATED PROBLEMS
  REVISE SOAP

in a person who is not exercising and eating well. By listing it as a potential problem, we are reminded to take measures to prevent it. This is a perfect use for the anticipated problem list.

Even in more complicated cases, where a patient may have more than one problem, the format remains the same. Under A (Assessment) we would list the problems in order of priority and be sure that we have a plan for each one. By checking each problem for a plan, and each plan for a problem, we can avoid missing anything. We can also avoid the very human practice of making plans for problems that don't exist.

3

BASIC
LIFE SUPPORT

Discussing serious problems first has its drawbacks. One can get the feeling that every accident is going to produce some tragic and overwhelming injury. It can make you a bit shy about taking risks or even letting yourself get more than a mile or two from a Level I trauma center. So please keep in mind that we cover the big problems first because they're big, not because they're common.

BASIC LIFE SUPPORT

Basic Life Support is the avenue of treatment pursued when confronting life-threatening major body system problems discovered during the Initial Assessment. The goal is to support oxygenation and perfusion of the vital organs while the patient assessment continues. In order for BLS to be effective, it must begin immediately at the scene.

In terms of saving lives, all BLS components are equally important. Although BLS is outlined in a specific sequence, field treatment requires flexibility. It is often necessary to change the order in which things are done, or to manage several components at the same time.

Most, but not all, of the procedures effective in Basic Life Support are covered by the obstructed airway and cardiopulmonary resuscitation (CPR) courses taught by the American Heart Association. We strongly recommend your participation in one of these courses, although you will no doubt have to adapt what you learn there to the wilderness environment.

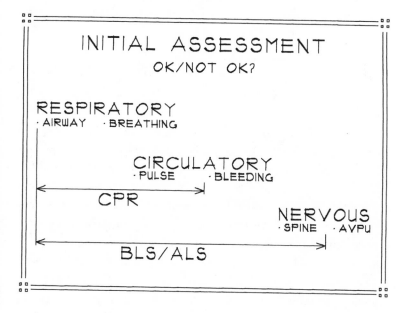

INITIAL ASSESSMENT
OK/NOT OK?

RESPIRATORY
· AIRWAY   · BREATHING

CIRCULATORY
· PULSE   · BLEEDING

CPR

NERVOUS
· SPINE   · AVPU

BLS/ALS

INITIAL ASSESSMENT

You'll remember from Chapter 2 and the Patient Assessment System that the Initial Assessment is a rapid check on the function of the circulatory, respiratory, and nervous systems. The easiest way to accomplish this is to ask the patient, "Hey, how are you?" If he gives an appropriate verbal response such as, "Ok, but my ankle is trapped under this log," you can be satisfied that there is no immediate life-threatening major system problem. He is breathing, his heart is beating, and his brain is functioning. You have done your Initial Assessment. In cases where the patient is unable to respond or has responded abnormally, you will need to look a little more closely.

BASIC LIFE SUPPORT—RESPIRATORY SYSTEM

RESPIRATORY DISTRESS

Is your patient moving enough air in and out to oxygenate her blood? If not, the cause may be airway obstruction, loss of nervous system control, chest-wall trauma, or swelling in the lungs or airway tubes. For the Initial Assessment it makes no difference—the issue is the same:

> Adequate ventilation means breathing OK
>
> Inadequate ventilation means breathing not OK

"Not OK" and "inadequate" are inexact terms for ventilation that is absent, too slow, or too shallow. If your patient is conscious, talk to her. A person who is able to speak generally has ventilation adequate for the Initial Assessment. A patient who can carry on a conversation is in pretty good shape from a respiratory point of view.

When respiratory distress is severe, conversation may be difficult or impossible. Light-skinned people may turn pale or blue. If you are unsure of respiratory status, the best criterion to use is your common sense. If you don't think your patient is breathing well enough, she most likely isn't. This is reason enough to begin to support ventilation with mouth-to-mouth or mouth-to-mask.

Inadequate or absent ventilation is treated by blowing into the lungs through the airway. This is called positive pressure ventilation (PPV). The rate of PPV should be about twelve breaths per minute (one every five seconds) or faster. If you don't like counting, just start the next breath as soon as the patient has finished exhaling. Blow in enough air to cause the chest to rise slightly. Each breath is done slowly over one to two seconds. Faster flow rates tend to blow air into the stomach, causing distension and vomiting.

Patients who are breathing on their own but not deeply or frequently enough can be assisted with ventilation timed to blow air in with the patient's own inspirations. This is especially useful in treating patients having difficulty breathing because of a chest-wall injury. Even if you can't time your ventilation exactly, a patient in trouble will quickly adjust to your efforts.

AIRWAY OBSTRUCTION AND AIRWAY OPENING TECHNIQUES

If you are unable to get air into the patient's lungs, the problem may be upper-airway obstruction. You may have already picked up some "foreign body in the airway" clues in your Scene Size-up: dinner time, steak and potatoes, the patient clutching her neck, that sort of thing. Other causes of obstruction include swelling, spasm, body position, and deformity from trauma.

Clearing an airway obstruction involves a progression of actions from the most simple to the most desperate. Because spine stabilization is a component of BLS, try not to move the patient's neck if injury is suspected. The airway is opened by a jaw thrust, chin lift, or a direct pull on the tongue while the patient's neck is held in the in-line position to protect the spinal cord. Beware of hyperextension of the neck (bending it back), which is frequently taught as an airway-opening technique. It helps very little and can be extremely harmful if the spine is injured.

"IN-LINE POSITION"

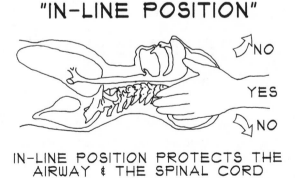

IN-LINE POSITION PROTECTS THE AIRWAY & THE SPINAL CORD

If this simple type of positioning does not open the airway, you must try to clear the obstruction manually. It is a perfectly natural reaction to want to look inside the mouth to figure out what's wrong.

Go ahead—you may see a foreign body that can be pulled out with your fingers or a clamp. Otherwise, try using gravity to clear obstructions. The usual method is to roll the patient's body to one side, keeping the spine in line, and "finger sweep" the mouth. If there is no reason to suspect spine injury, you can also roll the patient to a prone position and pull him up at the waist. This technique is especially effective in clearing vomit. In either position, a firm back blow between the shoulder blades can also help dislodge the obstruction.

Another way of clearing an obstruction is to place the patient on his or her back and give a sudden thrust to the abdomen or chest; this might possibly force out the air left in the patient's lungs, bringing with it anything blocking the airway. When an obstructed patient is still conscious and standing, this abdominal or chest thrust is done from behind by placing your own arms around the patient and squeezing. In either case, it really doesn't matter whether you are squeezing the abdomen or the chest in order for this method to be effective.

If the obstruction is due to swelling of the airway instead of a foreign body, back blows and abdominal thrusts will not help. Your best treatment will be to continue PPV in an attempt to force air past the obstruction while repositioning the neck for the best air flow. These patients will often need a "surgical airway" established by cutting directly into the trachea through the neck, which is an Advanced Life Support procedure.

BASIC LIFE SUPPORT—CIRCULATORY SYSTEM

CARDIAC ARREST

Cardiac arrest means the loss of effective heart contractions. In your Initial Assessment you check for the presence or absence of a pulse. Because cardiac arrest immediately causes respiratory arrest and complete loss of consciousness, *a patient who is at all responsive (A, V, and P on the AVPU scale), breathing, or moving spontaneously is not in cardiac arrest.*

> Pulse means circulation OK
>
> No pulse means circulation not OK

Although the pulse can be very difficult to find under adverse field conditions, weak or absent in the extremities of a person in shock, and very slow in profound hypothermia, it is extremely important to take the time to find it. The carotid and temporal pulses are the easiest to get to and are always present if the heart is beating. The carotid pulse is located on either side of the Adam's apple (larynx) in the neck. The temporal pulse is on either side of the head just in front of the ear.

Cardiac arrest is treated temporarily with cardiopulmonary resuscitation, which is a combination of chest compressions and ventilation (PPV) that allows some oxygenation and perfusion of the brain and vital organs. As outlined by the American Heart Association, CPR has been learned by millions of people and has saved many lives in settings where Advanced Life Support (ALS) is available within a few minutes.

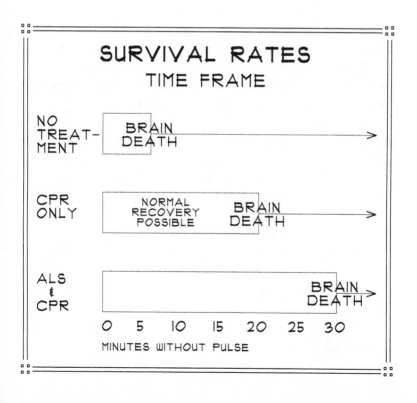

Unfortunately, CPR has very limited application in the backcountry. A patient has little chance of surviving unless his natural heart activity is restored within a short time, something that is extremely difficult to achieve without ALS with drugs and electrical defibrillation. Although ventilation can support breathing for hours or days, chest compressions cannot support perfusion of vital organs for long. In fact, the chances of survival are near zero if spontaneous heart activity is not restored within about thirty minutes. There may be exceptions to this in cases of severe hypothermia and cold-water drowning.

CPR will not restore life in situations where cardiac arrest is the result of massive trauma to the chest, severe blood loss, spinal cord transection, or head injury. In these cases it is best to realize that the patient has died. It is not useful to start or continue CPR when these conditions are discovered.

S E V E R E   B L E E D I N G

Adequate perfusion requires adequate circulating blood volume. Severe blood loss must be controlled as part of the BLS process. Always look carefully, for bleeding can be sometimes difficult to spot. It can be internal and hidden, but even profuse external bleeding can be missed. This is especially true with snow and bulky clothing, which can absorb or obscure blood. Exams can be troublesome when the patient's clothing is waterproof and the weather is too extreme to permit undressing.

Of all the forms of external bleeding, that coming from an artery is the most immediately life threatening. It will be under pressure and may spurt with the pulsing of the heart. Because there is no definite way to decide when bleeding is severe, the best rule of thumb might be: If it looks like a lot of blood, it probably is.

External bleeding is controlled by well-aimed direct pressure over the bleeding site. Pressure can be applied with a gloved hand if necessary, but a bandage or cloth should be used. This is not so much to absorb blood as to provide even pressure across the damaged vessels.

If bleeding continues, remove the bandage and look again for the source of blood, then re-aim your pressure. You should expect to apply pressure for fifteen or more minutes before a clot will form. Once bleeding is controlled, a pressure bandage should be applied. Beware, however, of obstructing circulation by creating an accidental tourniquet.

A tourniquet is applied only when you want to completely obstruct circulation to a limb. However, because you might be sacrificing the limb to save the life, it should be used only when there is no other way to stop bleeding, or when there is no time to do so. This may be necessary in mass-casualty disasters and in unstable and dangerous situations such as fire fighting or combat.

Unfortunately, internal bleeding is much harder to detect. It should always be suspected with a history of trauma and the development of shock. Severe internal bleeding is usually associated with fractures of the femur and pelvis and blunt abdominal and chest injury and is indicated by pain and the onset of volume shock. It is difficult to control without surgery. Even with the immediate availability of surgeons and operating rooms success is often limited. Severe internal bleeding in a wilderness setting is likely to be fatal. Less severe internal bleeding may be detected by the changes in vital signs as the body compensates for the loss of blood. In this case, immediate evacuation may be life saving.

BASIC LIFE SUPPORT—NERVOUS SYSTEM

SPINE INJURY

Injuries to the vertebral bones of the spinal column can damage the spinal cord with dramatic, devastating, and permanent results. This is why the stabilization of potential spine injury is considered part of Basic Life Support. The most dangerous movement of the cervical spine is flexion (movement of the chin toward the chest). Hyperextension (tilting the head back) is dangerous as well. Moderate extension is usually safe.

Any event that could produce spine injury, called a "positive mechanism," should be determined during your Scene Size-up. Examples include a fall from a cliff, being tumbled by an avalanche, or a short swim over a long waterfall. A determination of a positive mechanism means the patient should be treated as having spine injuries during the Initial Assessment. No further spine exam is necessary.

If no movement of the spine is required for lifesaving treatment, leave the patient where she is while you complete your assessment. If you must move the spine, bring the head and neck into the neutral (eyes forward) position in relation to the shoulders and chest. Stabilize the head and neck in this position during Basic Life Support and the rest of the patient survey. Spine splints, if necessary, are applied after the PAS is finished.

The airway can usually be kept clear of obstruction with the neck held in the neutral position. If it is necessary to roll the patient to clear vomit, roll the patient's body to the side with the head, neck, and trunk held in line as a unit. This can be tough to do if you are all by yourself. If you have to make a choice between a perfectly stable spine or an open airway, treat the airway. The benefits of breathing certainly outweigh the risks of spine injury.

LEVEL OF CONSCIOUSNESS

Reduced level of consciousness (V, P, and U on the AVPU scale) can be caused by severe nervous system injury or by loss of brain perfusion and oxygenation due to circulatory or respiratory system problems. There is no real way to treat reduced consciousness other than to treat the cause. Basic Life Support is aimed at protecting the airway from fluids and vomit and the spine from further injury while assessment and treatment continues. (By the way, using ammonia salts under the nose is not considered treatment.)

SECTION II

The Major

Body Systems

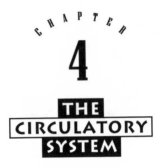

4

THE CIRCULATORY SYSTEM

To perfuse the body tissues with oxygenated blood, the circulatory system requires adequate pumping action from the heart, an intact system of vessels, and proper vessel constriction to maintain perfusion pressure. It also requires a sufficient volume of blood. To complete its part in the major system triad, the circulatory system must have oxygen faithfully supplied to the lungs by the respiratory system as well as good nervous system control of heart rate and blood vessel pressure.

There are three major components of the circulatory system.

1. *Heart* maintains blood flow and pressure through pumping action.
2. *Blood vessels* contain blood volume. Help maintain pressure through constriction controlled by nervous system.
3. *Blood* is the mixture of water, cells, and protein contained within circulatory system.

Normal circulatory system function requires:

1. Adequate pumping action from the heart

2. Integrity and constricting ability of blood vessels

3. Adequate volume of blood

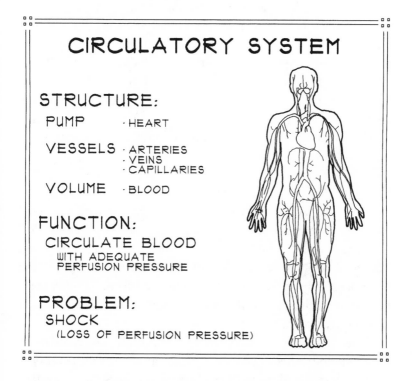

CIRCULATORY SYSTEM

STRUCTURE:

PUMP   · HEART

VESSELS · ARTERIES
         · VEINS
         · CAPILLARIES

VOLUME · BLOOD

FUNCTION:

CIRCULATE BLOOD
    WITH ADEQUATE
PERFUSION PRESSURE

PROBLEM:

SHOCK
    (LOSS OF PERFUSION PRESSURE)

CIRCULATORY SYSTEM PROBLEMS—SHOCK AND ACUTE STRESS REACTION

SHOCK

The term "shock" is often misunderstood and misrepresented. True shock is *not* caused by fatigue, disappointment, surprise, pain, grief, or any other reaction to *psychological* stress. These factors often cause Acute Stress Reaction, which can look like shock but has none of the serious consequences.

True shock is a *physiologic* condition, the acute loss of perfusion pressure in the circulatory system. Shock can be the result of failure of the pumping action of the heart due to trauma or heart attack (cardiogenic shock); of failure of blood vessel constriction due to anaphylaxis, infection, or spinal injury (vascular shock); or of loss of circulating blood volume due to bleeding or dehydration (volume shock). True shock always indicates a life-threatening physical condition that requires specific, aggressive treatment, preferably in the hospital. Without treatment, the patient will die.

Shock develops along a spectrum, from mild to severe. Progression can be stopped at any given point, but it is more common for shock to go from bad to worse. Of the various types of shock, the most commonly encountered in backcountry emergencies is volume shock from bleeding or dehydration.

ASSESSMENT OF VOLUME SHOCK.

A history of trauma sufficient to cause severe internal or external bleeding should make you think immediately of volume shock. This is also true of severe fluid loss from diarrhea, vomiting, or sweating. Volume shock's classic signs of cool and pale skin, rapid pulse, and rapid breathing are caused by the shell/core effect and other compensation mechanisms as the body attempts to maintain perfusion and oxygenation to the vital organs.

The vital-sign pattern reveals the compensation mechanisms at work, and the degree of change in vital signs reflects the severity of the fluid loss. The first vital-sign change to occur as shock develops is an increase in pulse rate followed closely by an increase in the respiratory rate. If you are able to measure blood pressure, you will observe that the compensatory mechanisms will keep it near normal in the early stages (compensated volume shock).

Compensation may work so well that it prevents symptoms from being noticed. As long as the oxygenation and perfusion of the brain is adequate, the patient's consciousness and mental status will be fairly normal. Unless you look carefully for compensation mechanisms at work and subtle changes in mental status, you may fail to recognize shock while there is still time to do something about it.

As the compensation mechanisms are overwhelmed, oxygenation and perfusion of the brain will be reduced, and the "evolutionary onion" will really start to peel. Mental status changes and other symptoms become more obvious as shock progresses. Ultimately, compensation will fail, perfusion pressure will fall, and level of consciousness will drop.

In a long-term-care situation, measuring urine output is another good way to monitor the status of the circulatory system. Reduced blood volume will result in greatly reduced urine output as the kidneys do their part to preserve fluid. This is an important sign to watch when you're concerned about the slow loss of fluid with burns, vomiting and diarrhea, and other forms of dehydration.

TREATMENT OF VOLUME SHOCK.

Shock from bleeding is a serious major body system problem that one cannot treat effectively in the backcountry. The traditional "treatments" of reassurance, elevating the feet, and keeping the patient warm are certainly good for anyone in shock but do nothing to

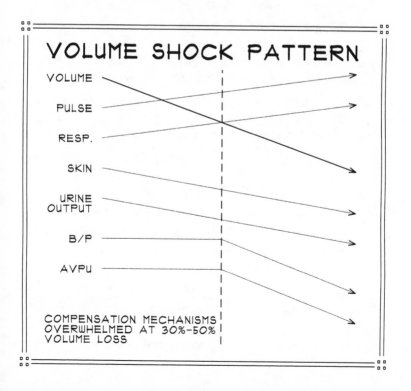

address the real problem of low blood volume. These are just temporary measures that may help stabilize the situation long enough to reach medical care. The patient needs intravenous (IV) fluids, surgeons, and a hospital. Volume shock is a true emergency, and you are justified in recruiting whatever help is necessary to get the patient to Advanced Life Support.

In the less urgent case of volume shock from slow dehydration (sweating, diarrhea), oral fluid replacement in the field may be sufficient if the shock is mild and you can stop the fluid losses.

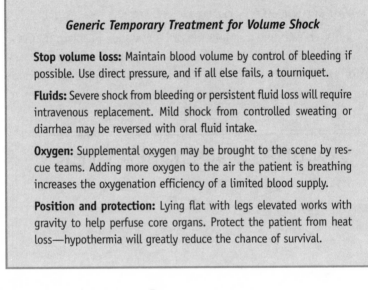

Generic Temporary Treatment for Volume Shock

Stop volume loss: Maintain blood volume by control of bleeding if possible. Use direct pressure, and if all else fails, a tourniquet.

Fluids: Severe shock from bleeding or persistent fluid loss will require intravenous replacement. Mild shock from controlled sweating or diarrhea may be reversed with oral fluid intake.

Oxygen: Supplemental oxygen may be brought to the scene by rescue teams. Adding more oxygen to the air the patient is breathing increases the oxygenation efficiency of a limited blood supply.

Position and protection: Lying flat with legs elevated works with gravity to help perfuse core organs. Protect the patient from heat loss—hypothermia will greatly reduce the chance of survival.

ACUTE STRESS REACTION

ASR is a frequent and normal response to physical and emotional stress of any type. Although this reaction can coexist with real life-threatening problems, it is more common for ASR to be a short-lived condition associated with minor injury.

Because Acute Stress Reaction is under the control of the nervous system, its symptoms may appear similar to true shock. However, the use of the term "psychogenic shock" for this phenomenon can be confusing and misleading because the consequences are very different from those of true shock. It is important to distinguish true shock, in its various degrees of compensation and levels of severity, from an acute stress reaction, which is not at all life threatening.

In the ambulance setting the difference is less important because both conditions are managed as shock during the short period of treatment and transport. For long-term management in the wilderness, however, recognizing ASR for what it is can save a lot of emergency resources, not to mention your piece of mind.

ASR comes in two basic forms:

1. ASR—SYMPATHETIC NERVOUS SYSTEM RESPONSE.

This is the "speed-up" response you feel when you're anxious or scared, produced by the release of the hormone adrenaline (epinephrine). Its effects increase the pulse and respiratory rate, shunt blood to the muscles, dilate the pupils, and generally get the body ready for action. Adrenaline also stimulates the release of natural hormones, which serves to mask the pain of injury.

This type of ASR certainly has value to human survival. It allows extraordinary efforts even in the presence of severe injury or other stress. Unfortunately, it also makes the accurate assessment of injuries difficult for the rescuer by hiding pain and altering vital signs.

2. ASR—PARASYMPATHETIC NERVOUS SYSTEM RESPONSE.

Feeling faint and nauseated in response to stress is another familiar feeling. It is caused by a temporary loss of perfusion of the brain due to a sudden slowing of the heart rate. The evolutionary value of this response is difficult to figure out. This condition too is physiologically harmless except in its ability to mimic the shell/core effect seen in true volume shock.

ASSESSMENT OF ASR.

The key to recognizing Acute Stress Reaction is in the mechanism of injury and the progression of symptoms. ASR can look like shock but can occur with or without any mechanism of injury that can cause shock. With time ASR will get better, especially if your treatment reduces pain and anxiety.

We have all seen people with only minor extremity sprains or superficial wounds become light-headed, pale, and nauseated. Although they look "shocky," there is no cause for alarm, and certainly no need for helicopters and emergency surgery. Usually, if there is no mechanism for sudden volume loss, you can assume any shock-like symptoms can be attributed to ASR.

It is important to remember that Acute Stress Reaction can coexist with shock. In cases where the patient has both a mechanism of injury for true shock and the signs and symptoms to go with it, you must treat it as such.

FIELD TREATMENT OF ASR.

Allowing the patient to lie down, providing calm reassurance, and relieving pain by treating injuries should result in immediate improvement in symptoms. Note that this is the traditional treatment for shock described in many first-aid texts.

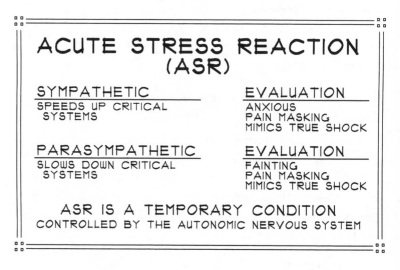

ACUTE STRESS REACTION (ASR)

SYMPATHETIC
SPEEDS UP CRITICAL
SYSTEMS

EVALUATION
ANXIOUS
PAIN MASKING
MIMICS TRUE SHOCK

PARASYMPATHETIC
SLOWS DOWN CRITICAL
SYSTEMS

EVALUATION
FAINTING
PAIN MASKING
MIMICS TRUE SHOCK

ASR IS A TEMPORARY CONDITION
CONTROLLED BY THE AUTONOMIC NERVOUS SYSTEM

Case Study—Circulatory System

S: An eighteen-year-old man skiing out of bounds fell against a stump, injuring his right upper leg, and is unable to move without extreme pain. He reports feeling a little chilled but has not been shivering. He can feel and wiggle the toes in his right boot. The patient has no other complaints.

   The friend who reported the accident described a tumbling fall through the trees. There was no loss of consciousness. The ski patroller who found the patient noted that the path of his fall was about sixty feet through rocks and stumps. The air temperature was 22 degrees Fahrenheit with a moderate north wind. It was 11:00 in the morning. All skiers in the party were accounted for.

O: Ski patrollers found the patient lying in a stable position on his back in the snow. The patient was found to be alert and oriented but anxious and uncomfortable. He remembered the whole event.

   Exam revealed a tender and swollen right thigh. There were no other major injuries found. There was no external bleeding found inside the ski clothing. Vital signs at 11:30: BP: unknown; P: 120; R: 32; C: A on AVPU scale, anxious; Skin: pale and cool; T: unknown.

A: 1. Compensated volume shock from bleeding into the thigh

    2. Fracture R thigh

    3. Cold environment

    4. Acute Stress Reaction

A': 1. Severe shock

    2. Distal ischemia R leg

    3. Hypothermia

P: 1. Immediate evacuation to advanced life support

    2. Splint thigh by immobilizing patient in toboggan

    3. Hypothermia wrap and transport

    4. Relieve pain and anxiety through treatment and reassurance

Discussion: This patient presents a couple of different problems common to the backcountry. He certainly has a positive mechanism for shock, and his vital-sign pattern confirms it. He also has a bit of ASR, which one would expect with a broken leg. The cold environment and immobility of the patient adds the *anticipated* problem of hypothermia.

CIRCULATORY SYSTEM SUMMARY

PROBLEM	EVALUATION	TREATMENT
VOLUME SHOCK	BLEEDING & VS PATTERN OF SHOCK	STOP BLEEDING IV FLUIDS OXYGEN POSITION & PROTECT EVACUATE
VOLUME SHOCK	SEVERE DEHYDRATION & VS PATTERN OF SHOCK	STOP FLUID LOSS IV FLUIDS OXYGEN POSITION & PROTECT EVACUATE
VOLUME SHOCK	MILD DEHYDRATION & VS PATTERN FOR COMPENSATED SHOCK	STOP FLUID LOSS ORAL FLUIDS OXYGEN POSITION & PROTECT MONITOR EVACUATE IF NOT IMPROVING

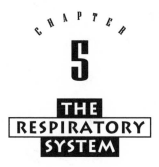

CHAPTER 5

THE RESPIRATORY SYSTEM

The respiratory system performs the task of bringing oxygen to the blood and removing carbon dioxide. The exchange takes place in the alveoli of the lungs, where only a thin semipermeable membrane separates the outside air from the blood. The rest of the system consists of semirigid tubes to conduct air to the alveoli and a bellows system composed of the chest wall and muscles for moving the air in and out.

Like the circulatory system, the respiratory system is under nervous system control. In a healthy patient, breathing is controlled by the brain as it measures the pH (acidity) of the blood (which is actually a reflection of the amount of dissolved carbon dioxide it contains). Too much carbon dioxide in the blood causes acidity to increase. The brain responds by increasing the rate and depth of respiration to "blow off" the carbon dioxide until a normal pH is reestablished. Conversely, too little carbon dioxide is corrected by decreasing the rate and depth of respiration.

This carbon dioxide regulation system is very precise, and it results in a smooth and regular respiratory pattern. But in some

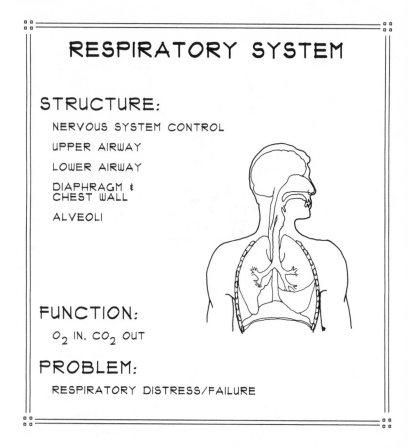

RESPIRATORY SYSTEM

STRUCTURE:

NERVOUS SYSTEM CONTROL

UPPER AIRWAY

LOWER AIRWAY

DIAPHRAGM &
CHEST WALL

ALVEOLI

FUNCTION:

O_2 IN, CO_2 OUT

PROBLEM:

RESPIRATORY DISTRESS/FAILURE

disease conditions, like emphysema, the amount of carbon dioxide in the blood is high all the time because the lungs are damaged and cannot function properly. The brain then falls back on measuring the amount of oxygen in the blood to determine breathing rate and depth. This process is much less precise, is more easily upset, and results in a more irregular breathing pattern.

There are five major components of the respiratory system:

1. *Upper airway* consists of the mouth (oropharynx), nose (nasopharynx), and throat (larynx).

2. *Lower airway* is composed of large tubes (trachea), smaller tubes (bronchi), and the smallest tubes (bronchioles).

3. *Alveoli* are the membranous air sacs at the end of the system adjacent to blood-filled capillaries where oxygen and carbon dioxide exchange occurs.

4. *Chest wall/diaphragm.* In normal function, this operates much like a bellows. Inspiration (the intake of air) is caused by the active contraction of the diaphragm and chest-wall muscles; this allows the chest cavity to expand and suck air into the lungs. Expiration (air out) is a passive process that occurs when these muscles relax and the natural elasticity of the lungs and chest squeeze out the air.

5. *Nervous system control.* The nervous system (brain) controls the rate and depth of respiration in response to the amount of carbon dioxide and oxygen in the blood.

Normal respiratory system function requires:

1. Open upper airway

2. Open lower airway

3. Alveoli with membrane exposed to air

4. Functioning "bellows" mechanism

5. Intact nervous system

RESPIRATORY SYSTEM PROBLEMS

"Respiratory distress" is the generic term for dozens of different problems that can develop directly in the respiratory system or indirectly as a result of circulatory or nervous system problems. These problems all produce the same generic symptoms, including increased respiratory rate, increased respiratory effort, and noise (wheeze, cough, stridor). All have the same generic effect: reduced oxygen supply to the blood. We can condense these problems into five broad categories, which are given the same generic treatment, with a few additional specifics (because the generic treatment applies to all respiratory problems, we'll outline it first so you can take it with you as you read the rest of the section).

Generic Treatment for Respiratory Distress

Position. Any patient in respiratory distress who is able to move will have found the best position in which to breathe. This is usually sitting up to allow gravity to assist the diaphragm and to help keep fluids out of the airway tubes. In unconscious or immobile patients, special care must be taken to position them in a way that prevents airway obstruction from secretions, vomit, or the collapse of their own airways. This is usually on the side, with the head and neck in the "in-line" position.

Reassurance. Encourage the patient to breathe slower and deeper rather than pant like a dog. This brings in fresh oxygen instead of moving the same old carbon dioxide back and forth in the tubes.

Ventilation. A patient in respiratory distress will fatigue rapidly. You may need to provide positive pressure ventilation to assist the patient's efforts. This PPV, produced by the rescuer blowing air in as the patient tries to inhale, can often work where the patient cannot draw air in on her own.

Oxygen. If it is available, supplemental oxygen will increase the concentration of oxygen getting into the blood, and ultimately to the brain.

UPPER AIRWAY OBSTRUCTION

The upper airway may be obstructed by the tongue, a piece of food, or even as a result of the patient's head being under water. Obstruction can also develop slowly with swelling from trauma or infection.

ASSESSMENT OF AIRWAY OBSTRUCTION.

If the Initial Assessment reveals the absence of respiration, even if the patient is still conscious, Basic Life Support must begin immediately (see Chapter 3).

If airway obstruction is not complete, the patient may have noisy and difficult respiration. The term *stridor* is used to describe the stuttering sound made by inhalation against an upper-airway obstruction. The ability to swallow is often impaired, and the patient may be drooling. Talking may be difficult or impossible.

When dealing with partial obstruction, it is important to determine whether the patient is getting enough air to support life until medical care can be reached. Look for signs that oxygenation of the blood is adequate: good skin color, awake (A on the AVPU scale), and no worsening of the respiratory distress.

TREATMENT OF AIRWAY OBSTRUCTION.

For the treatment of complete airway obstruction or partial obstruction with inadequate oxygenation, refer to Basic Life Support (Chapter 3).

In cases where a foreign object is lodged in the throat for a brief time and successfully removed before the patient gets in real trouble, you may certainly congratulate yourself on a real "save." However, the object may have caused enough irritation of the airway to result in the development of obstruction from swelling, and this should be on your anticipated problem list for the next twenty-four hours.

In cases of partial airway obstruction with adequate oxygenation, the rule is "do no harm." Apply the generic treatment for respiratory distress and evacuate quickly. In almost all cases of partial obstruction, breathing cool air will reduce swelling of the airway temporarily. Also keep in mind that a partial obstruction frequently becomes worse over time. Be prepared to perform opening maneuvers if it becomes apparent that the airway is closing.

LOWER AIRWAY CONSTRICTION

Spasm, swelling, or the accumulation of mucus or pus can cause narrowing of the lower airway tubes (bronchi and bronchioles). This is what happens in asthma, bronchitis, and anaphylaxis. The effect is to slow the movement of air in and out of the alveoli.

ASSESSMENT OF LOWER AIRWAY CONSTRICTION.

Expiration is often prolonged, with wheezing and gurgling. Sometimes the lower airway noise is loud enough to hear from a distance. Other times you may need a stethoscope or an ear to the patient's chest to detect a lower airway constriction.

The patient may describe exposure to smoke, inhalation of water, or some other irritating substance, indicating a generalized swelling. He may have been exposed to something to which he is allergic, indicating anaphylaxis. Or there may be a history of slowly worsening illness and fever pointing to respiratory infection. Whatever the cause, the patient usually develops a cough as the respiratory system tries to clear itself. There may be an obvious increase in respiratory effort as the system struggles to move air against increased resistance. Vital signs may show increases in the compensatory mechanisms, with elevated heart and respiratory rates.

Treatment of Lower Airway Constriction.

1. Generic treatment for respiratory distress.
2. Specific treatment for lower airway constriction: Treatment with antibiotics for infection, and/or bronchodilators (usually given as a spray inhaler) for asthma may be necessary. In the presence of respiratory distress, emergency evacuation is appropriate.

Pulmonary Edema

With pulmonary edema, excess fluid accumulates in the alveoli, blocking the exchange of oxygen and carbon dioxide between air and blood. This fluid usually comes from within the body as capillaries leak into the alveoli, often as a result of too much pressure in part of the circulatory system (for example, from congestive heart failure, swelling in reaction to irritants like water or smoke, or as part of the effect of reduced oxygen at high altitude). Also, a contusion or laceration of the lung tissue may cause the alveoli to fill with blood. In other cases, the inflammation from infection, such as pneumonia, can fill the alveoli with pus.

Assessment of Pulmonary Edema.

Large amounts of fluid in the lungs will cause gurgling that can be heard at a distance. Fluid may actually froth at the mouth ("talking in bubbles"). Small amounts of fluid may be detected by putting an ear to the chest and listening for "crackling" sounds on respiration. Vital signs will show that the body is compensating for partial loss of lung function with an increase in respiratory and heart rates. The development of fever indicates infection.

In less severe cases, reduced lung function may be noticeable only when the patient is exerting himself. With the increased demands of exercise reduced lung capacity will become obvious, for the patient becomes short of breath much more easily than would be normal.

Coughing is common with the accumulation of pulmonary fluid, and sometimes the patient may cough up sputum tinged with pus or blood. There may be a history of injury to lung tissue through exposure to smoke, infection, or near drowning. Or, you may have just climbed above 12,000 feet on your way to the top of a 14,000-foot mountain and are experiencing the beginning of high altitude pulmonary edema (HAPE).

TREATMENT OF PULMONARY EDEMA

1. Generic treatment for respiratory distress.
2. Specific treatment for pulmonary fluid: Evacuation to medical care. Antibiotics for suspected pneumonia. In high altitude sickness, immediate descent to a lower altitude.

CHEST TRAUMA

Trauma to the chest wall or airway tubes can interfere with the function of the respiratory system in a number of ways. Because chest trauma with respiratory distress is often complicated and severe and cannot be effectively managed in the field, it is best to evacuate the patient without delay.

"Lung contusion" is the term applied to the development of swelling in lung tissue following injury. The chest wall may still be stable, but pulmonary fluid begins to accumulate in the alveoli. This should be an anticipated problem with suspected rib fracture or any severe blow to the chest. As a rough guide, "getting the wind knocked out of you" is severe enough to warrant suspicion of significant chest trauma.

An unstable chest wall, also called a "flail chest," indicates that the bellows system is damaged to the point that it is no longer rigid. Instead of the lungs expanding with inspiration, the chest wall collapses.

Hemothorax and *pneumothorax* are terms used to describe the presence of blood (heme) or air (pneumo) in the chest cavity (thorax). This blood or air occupies the space between the lungs and the chest wall, preventing full expansion of the lungs, shifting the heart out of position, and putting pressure on the great vessels of the chest. In the case of an open pneumothorax, sometimes called a "sucking chest wound," air may enter the chest cavity through an injury in the chest wall. In a closed pneumothorax, air may enter the chest cavity through an injured lung. It may affect only one side of the chest or both.

ASSESSMENT OF CHEST TRAUMA.

There will be a history of significant blunt trauma to the chest or evidence of penetrating injury. There may be bruising, fractured ribs, or other evidence of potential injury to lungs or the chest wall. It will be apparent by level of consciousness and mental status changes and other vital signs that the patient is not getting enough oxygen. Significant injury to the circulatory system also often occurs with severe chest trauma and will result in volume shock.

TREATMENT OF CHEST TRAUMA

1. Generic treatment for respiratory distress. Like the treatment for shock, this is limited and temporary only. The patient with chest injury significant enough to cause respiratory distress deserves immediate evacuation.

2. Specific treatment for chest trauma: Having the patient lie on the injured side reduces pain by splinting the chest wall. Gravity can help keep blood from building up in the uninjured side of the chest.

In case of a simple rib fracture, reducing pain by helping the patient find a comfortable position and using pain medication will make breathing more comfortable and reduce respiratory distress. A tight rib belt, which is suggested by some first-aid texts, will restrict breathing and should be used with extreme caution, if at all.

In cases of open chest wounds with air passing in and out of the hole, the injury should be covered with an airtight seal, such as a piece of plastic bag. Don't worry about trying to make a one-way valve or coordinating the patch placement with inspiration. Just put it on. If applying a patch improves the situation, leave it in place. If symptoms become worse, remove it.

RESPIRATORY ARREST (LOSS OF NERVOUS SYSTEM CONTROL)

Breathing is controlled by the nervous system. If the nervous system is damaged, breathing may be irregular or slow. If the nervous system stops working, breathing will stop. Possible causes of respiratory arrest include toxins and drugs, head injury, altitude sickness, lightning strike, and hypothermia.

ASSESSMENT OF RESPIRATORY ARREST.

As respiratory drive decreases, respiratory rate and effort decreases, becomes irregular, or stops. The fact that respiration is inadequate is not always clear. Level of consciousness will already be reduced by the primary nervous system problem and therefore is not a reliable indicator. Anyone with slowed or irregular breathing and reduced consciousness should be considered in need of positive pressure ventilation and oxygen. Don't be timid about this: PPV carries a very low risk of causing harm and provides great benefit if the patient really needs it.

TREATMENT FOR RESPIRATORY ARREST

1. Basic Life Support.
2. Generic treatment for respiratory distress.
3. Correct the nervous system problem if possible. If not, evacuate.

HYPERVENTILATION (INCREASED RESPIRATORY DRIVE)

Increased respiratory drive occurs with altitude, exercise, injury, and illness. This is a normal response to physiologic demands, requiring more oxygen and producing more carbon dioxide. Increased respiration also occurs with Acute Stress Reaction, but not in response to an increased need for oxygen or excess production of carbon dioxide. The result of hyperventilation in ASR can be an abnormal decrease in the carbon dioxide concentration in the blood with the associated abnormal decrease in acidity. This is blood chemistry out of balance, which can produce a variety of nervous system symptoms that are referred to as hyperventilation syndrome.

ASSESSMENT OF HYPERVENTILATION.

Hyperventilation can occur with or without obvious fast and heavy breathing. It only takes a slight increase in depth and rate over time to cause changes in blood acidity. The respiratory changes observed in your measurement of vital signs may be very subtle.

It can be difficult to distinguish between hyperventilation syndrome and serious respiratory or nervous system problems, especially if there is a positive mechanism for injury. As with other components of Acute Stress Reaction, however, hyperventilation gets better with time and basic treatment.

There are some classic nervous system effects of hyperventilation worth mentioning. Tingling of the hands and feet and numbness around the mouth is common. The patient may feel paralyzed, but his or her ability to move is not actually impaired.

TREATMENT OF HYPERVENTILATION

1. Generic treatment for respiratory distress.

2. Specific Treatment for Hyperventilation Syndrome: Reducing stress is specific and effective. Patients generally feel better when given an explanation of their symptoms and can be coached to breathe slower and more regularly.

Case Study—Respiratory System

A backcountry ranger responded to the scene of an apparent illness on an Adirondack canoe portage. It was midmorning; the weather was partly cloudy with light winds and temperatures in the sixties. One member of a group of twelve teenagers was having trouble breathing. The rest of the group were all accounted for and in no trouble.

S: A thirteen-year-old boy with a history of asthma developed respiratory distress in the middle of a mile-long portage. Witnesses reported that he used his medication inhaler just before setting out but quickly became short of breath. He set his canoe on a tree and slumped to the ground. There was no history of trauma or insect stings. The boy had no allergies. He was taking no additional medications. Asthma had been diagnosed several years ago. He last ate at 0900. He had not been otherwise ill. The patient was working too hard to breathe to give any useful information.

O: Initial Assessment showed an awake but confused boy in obvious respiratory distress. Exam revealed no other injury.

Vital Signs at 11:00: P: 120; R: 40 with wheezing; BP: no BP cuff, but pulse was felt at the wrist; S: cool, pale, blue lips; T: felt cool, but core temperature probably OK; C: Awake, but confused and anxious.

A: Respiratory distress from lower-airway constriction (asthma)

A': Respiratory failure

P: The boy was assisted into a sitting position to help his breathing. Group members were sent to both ends of the portage to look for the boy's medication. Oxygen was not available, but the ranger was carrying a pocket mask to use for PPV if necessary.

The inhaled medication did not help. Evacuation was carried out by canoe to an ALS ambulance crew that had been called by radio. By the end of the trip the patient was V on AVPU, and positive pressure ventilation had been started. Following treatment with injectable medication in the ambulance and hospital, the boy improved quickly.

Discussion: With the history available from group members, the ranger could make the specific assessment of asthma and include the boy's medication in the plan. Without this information he would be left with the general diagnosis of respiratory distress due to lower-airway constriction. There could be several causes, but the treatment would be the same.

RESPIRATORY SYSTEM SUMMARY

PROBLEM	EVALUATION	TREATMENT
UPPER AIRWAY OBSTRUCTION	NO AIR IN OR OUT	GENERIC TREATMENT RELIEVE OBSTRUCTION
LOWER AIRWAY CONSTICTION	COUGHING WHEEZING RESPIRATORY DISTRESS	GENERIC TREATMENT MEDICATIONS EVACUATION
PULMONARY FLUIDS	COUGHING GURGLING RESPIRATORY DISTRESS	GENERIC TREATMENT MEDICATIONS DESCENT/ EVACUATION
CHEST TRAUMA	PAIN DEFORMITY BRUISING RESPIRATORY DISTRESS	GENERIC TREATMENT PAIN MEDS EVACUATION
RESPIRATORY FAILURE	ABSENT OR SLOW RESPIRATION	GENERIC TREATMENT EVACUATION

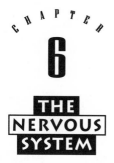

CHAPTER

6

THE NERVOUS SYSTEM

The nervous system consists of the brain, spinal cord, and peripheral nerves. The brain, in addition to being responsible for remembering where you left your flashlight, controls all critical life functions. Its primary connection with the circulatory and respiratory systems is through the spinal cord. Both the brain and spinal cord are encased within the bony structure of the skull and the vertebrae of the spine.

From the gap between vertebrae, peripheral nerves branch out from the spinal cord to all body tissues. Nerves controlling the most critical functions exit the cord at the base of the skull and in the neck. This is why spinal-cord injuries that occur in this area can cause extreme disability or death due to the loss of nervous system control over vital body functions.

All nervous system tissue is extremely sensitive to injury, especially oxygen deprivation. If the brain is involved, reduced oxygenation and perfusion will immediately affect mental status, giving one of the best first indicators of a developing life-threatening condition.

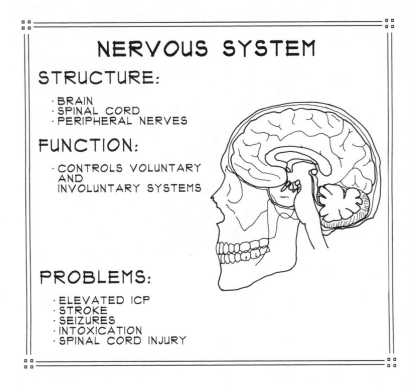

NERVOUS SYSTEM

STRUCTURE:

- BRAIN
- SPINAL CORD
- PERIPHERAL NERVES

FUNCTION:

- CONTROLS VOLUNTARY AND INVOLUNTARY SYSTEMS

PROBLEMS:

- ELEVATED ICP
- STROKE
- SEIZURES
- INTOXICATION
- SPINAL CORD INJURY

There are two major components of the nervous system.

1. *The central nervous system* consists of the brain and spinal cord encased in the bony protection of the skull and spine and bathed in cerebrospinal fluid.

2. *The peripheral nervous system* is composed of the unprotected nerves running between the central nervous system and the body tissues. These nerves typically occur in bundles along with arteries and veins.

Normal nervous system function requires:

1. Uninterrupted perfusion of the central nervous system with oxygenated blood.

2. Intact central and peripheral nerve pathways between the central nervous system and the body tissues.

NERVOUS SYSTEM PROBLEMS

INCREASED INTRACRANIAL PRESSURE (ICP)

The brain, like other body tissues, will swell from bleeding and edema when injured. However, the brain is confined within the rigid structure of the skull (cranium) so that when it swells there can be a dangerous rise in intracranial pressure. A severe head injury, stroke, or high altitude cerebral edema (HACE) can create such severe swelling that perfusion and oxygenation of brain tissue cannot take place.

ASSESSMENT OF INCREASED ICP.

Like shock, increased ICP has a typical pattern and spectrum of severity regardless of its cause or rate of onset.

History. Look for a mechanism of injury to brain tissue such as trauma, suffocation, or high altitude.

Vital signs. Although other vital-sign changes occur, alteration of consciousness and mental status is the most sensitive early indicator of increased ICP. This is the peeling of the evolutionary onion again. The patient may appear drunk or become combative or restless, quickly moving down the AVPU scale as ICP progresses. *It can be very difficult to tell the difference between someone who is intoxicated by alcohol or drugs and a patient with increased ICP.*

Vomiting. With a positive mechanism of injury, persistent vomiting is a reliable early sign of increasing ICP.

Headache. Severe headache is an early sign of increased ICP. However, it is easily confused with pain from an injured neck, scalp, or skull.

Unequal pupil dilation. This is a late sign in elevated ICP, developing only after the obvious changes in consciousness have already indicated a serious problem. It is worthy of mention here because it is frequently cited by rescuers as evidence of brain injury, even in patients showing no mental status changes. An alert, oriented person with unequal pupil dilation has an eye problem, or it is a normal physiological feature of the individual. Don't concentrate on this sign out of context.

Other signs. Paralysis, seizures, irregular breathing, or other signs of major body system problems may also develop late in the progress of ICP. They may follow consciousness and mental status changes by minutes, hours, or days.

TREATMENT OF INCREASED ICP.

Because surgery is generally required to relieve pressure and stop intracranial bleeding, field treatment will have little effect on the patient's chances for recovery. The rapid onset of severe swelling from intracranial bleeding will be fatal in most backcountry settings. Severe nervous system damage cannot be overcome with CPR.

On the other hand, the early recognition of swelling that may be developing more slowly can save lives. The key is good Basic Life Support and rapid evacuation with special attention to protection of the cervical spine and the airway. As long as there is a heartbeat, there is a chance of at least partial recovery.

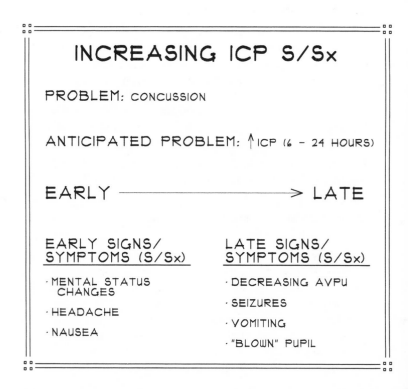

INCREASING ICP S/Sx

PROBLEM: CONCUSSION

ANTICIPATED PROBLEM: ↑ICP (6 – 24 HOURS)

EARLY ——————————> LATE

EARLY SIGNS/
SYMPTOMS (S/Sx)

· MENTAL STATUS
  CHANGES

· HEADACHE

· NAUSEA

LATE SIGNS/
SYMPTOMS (S/Sx)

· DECREASING AVPU

· SEIZURES

· VOMITING

· "BLOWN" PUPIL

Concussion (Minor Head Injury)

"Head injury," which refers specifically to an injury to the brain, is an often misused term. It is important to distinguish head injury, with its nervous system problems, from head wounds, such as injuries to the scalp or face, which do not involve brain injury.

Minor head injury, usually referred to as concussion, occurs when the patient strikes his head while falling, or when something falls on the patient's head. The event results in a temporary change in brain function, indicating that the brain has suffered some degree of injury, although ICP is not elevated.

Assessment of Minor Head Injury.

Typically, the patient experiences a brief loss of consciousness (V or P on the AVPU scale), sees "stars," or has a lapse of memory. There may be a short period of disorientation or loss of memory about the event itself ("What happened? How did I get here?"). He may feel dazed, sleepy, or nauseated. There is usually a mild to moderate headache that is easily treated with aspirin or ibuprofen.

The important question in a concussion is whether the injured brain tissue will swell enough in the subsequent twenty-four hours to cause a dangerous increase in intracranial pressure. Will this minor concussion become a severe head injury? This is one of the classic backcountry medical dilemmas: to evacuate now, or wait and watch.

There are no absolute rules, but there some general guidelines. Minor head injuries associated with the following red flags are more likely to become serious problems.

Red Flags for Minor Head Injury
Loss of consciousness at any time.

The exam shows any decline in consciousness or mental status following the event.

There is any deformity of the skull.

The patient vomits more than once, or complains of persistent severe headache.

The patient exhibits "antegrade amnesia," the progression of memory loss to include events occurring after the initial injury.

The patient may forget what has been happening from minute to minute as you talk to him. This symptom is worth special consideration because it can be pretty funny to witness. Don't laugh; take it very seriously.

TREATMENT OF MINOR HEAD INJURY.

Concussion requires no specific field treatment. However, it is important to monitor the patient carefully for at least twenty-four hours to detect the possible onset of increased ICP. Patients being monitored should not use narcotic or stimulant drugs or drink alcohol because this will confuse the assessment of consciousness and mental status. It is not necessary to keep a concussed patient awake. The pain and vomiting of increasing ICP will wake them quite effectively.

Generally, in a remote backcountry setting, it is best to begin planning for the evacuation of a patient with confirmed concussion rather than to wait for the onset of ICP. This is especially true of

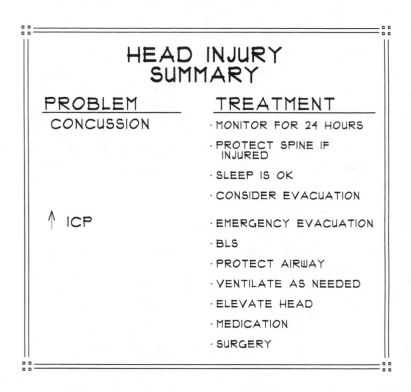

HEAD INJURY SUMMARY

PROBLEM	TREATMENT
CONCUSSION	· MONITOR FOR 24 HOURS
	· PROTECT SPINE IF INJURED
	· SLEEP IS OK
	· CONSIDER EVACUATION
↑ ICP	· EMERGENCY EVACUATION
	· BLS
	· PROTECT AIRWAY
	· VENTILATE AS NEEDED
	· ELEVATE HEAD
	· MEDICATION
	· SURGERY

patients with red flag signs and symptoms. We also must remember to evaluate and treat for cervical spine injury, which has the same mechanism of injury.

STROKE

A stroke is what the medical profession politely refers to as a "cerebral vascular accident," as if the brain didn't really mean to do it. The "accident" happens when a blood vessel inside the brain ruptures and bleeds, or a clot lodges in an artery. The initial effect of either event is ischemia and infarction, which may be very localized or very extensive. Elevated ICP may soon follow, especially with intracranial bleeding.

ASSESSMENT OF STROKE.

A sudden change in brain function without a history of trauma or intoxication should make you think of stroke. It may be as subtle as a little numbness in one hand or arm or a slight facial droop, or as dramatic as complete paralysis of one side of the body or the sudden loss of the ability to speak.

In some cases the symptoms are transient, resolving after a few minutes or hours as a clot forms and then dissolves. These transient ischemic attacks are a warning of permanent disability to come.

TREATMENT OF STROKE.

Stroke is an emergency, and the patient must be hospitalized. During evacuation, apply Basic Life Support and treat as you would any patient with existing or anticipated elevated ICP.

SEIZURES

Brain tissue has electrical properties much like heart tissue. Seizures are an uncoordinated burst of electrical activity in the brain brought about by a variety of causes.

ASSESSMENT OF SEIZURE.

In assessing a seizure it is important to consider the context in which it has occurred. Seizures can be part of the pattern of increased ICP in trauma patients or a relatively normal occurrence in a patient with epilepsy. They can be related to drug use or can occur for no apparent reason in an otherwise healthy individual.

The classic grand mal seizure is characterized by generalized tensing of all body muscles and repetitive, purposeless movement. Although the eyes may be open, the patient will be unresponsive during the seizure. He may be incontinent of feces and urine. There will usually be a period of drowsiness and disorientation after the seizure has ended.

TREATMENT OF SEIZURE.

Protection from injury is the most important treatment one can provide to a seizure patient. Most seizures will resolve spontaneously in a short period of time. Protect the patient from injury when she is falling or thrashing. Protect her also from unnecessary treatments like chest compressions or rescuers trying to force objects between her teeth.

Seizure patients will normally hold their breath briefly and become cyanotic (blue). This is not a problem as long as it does not last more than a couple of minutes. Position the patient and ventilate if necessary after the seizure has resolved, or during the seizure if you feel respirations are inadequate.

The real worry, of course, is not the seizure itself but what has caused it. Unless the patient is a known epileptic who has frequent seizures, the cause must be researched by a medical practitioner. Because a seizure may be the first sign of a serious condition, evacuation is a good idea. However, it is not an emergency situation if the seizure resolves spontaneously and the patient seems otherwise OK.

INTOXICATION

Intoxication refers to a change in brain function due to the effects of a foreign chemical, often taken intentionally. Alcohol and caffeine are common examples of intoxication, but there hundreds of others. In an emergency, the effects can be generally classified as depressant or stimulant. Depressants are the most dangerous intoxicants, especially when they reduce the nervous system's respiratory drive.

Assessment of Intoxication.

Your survey of the scene and history should clue you in to the mechanism of injury. If the intoxication is severe, with the patient below V on the AVPU scale, he will be at risk for airway obstruction and inadequate respiration. In less severe cases, the danger may be indirect, for instance, hypothermia, frostbite, or stumbling overboard.

Treatment of Intoxication.

Protect the airway from vomit, fluids, or mechanical obstruction. Give positive pressure ventilation if respiration seems inadequate. Protect the patient from heat loss. Evacuate if the intoxication is severe. Fortunately, most intoxicating chemicals will be metabolized and excreted by the body within a few hours.

Spinal Cord Trauma

The delicate tissue of the spinal cord, really an extension of the brain, is surrounded and protected by the bones of the spinal column. Unstable injuries of the spinal column, such as fracture or dislocation, can easily injure the cord. Spinal cord injuries are usually permanent, but recovery is sometimes possible with careful treatment.

Field Assessment and Treatment of Spinal Cord Injury.

This is essentially the same as that for spine fracture, which is discussed along with other fractures in Chapter 7. Even if the cord is already injured, careful extrication, treatment, and evacuation will control further damage and increase the chance of recovery.

Peripheral Nerves

The peripheral nervous system encompasses all nervous tissue outside of the brain and spinal cord. Peripheral nerves have the same cable-like structure as the spinal cord, but they are not encased in the same bony protection. This leaves them even more susceptible to contusion from direct impact, or laceration and tearing in fractures and dislocations.

Peripheral nerves are also affected by pressure, which can deprive them of adequate perfusion. "Backpacker's palsy" is the gradual onset of tingling and numbness in the arms caused by pressure on nerves in the armpit and shoulder, created by pack straps.

ASSESSMENT OF PERIPHERAL NERVE INJURY.

Loss of movement and sensation in the area beyond the site of an injury can indicate nerve damage, for which little can be done in the field. However, you will remember that this can be caused by ischemia (loss of blood circulation), which is usually easily remedied.

TREATMENT OF PERIPHERAL NERVE INJURY.

In the field, the treatment of peripheral nerve injury is the same as the treatment for loss of circulation. Both can be fixed by removing the source of pressure, for instance by loosening a splint, realigning a fracture or dislocation, or reducing the swelling of an injured extremity. This is generic fracture management and is discussed in Chapter 7.

Case Study—Nervous System

A forty-year-old fisherman was struck on the head while trying to secure a trawl door on a forty-seven-foot fishing vessel fifty miles offshore. The time was 04:30. The weather was clear with winds of 15 knots, three-foot waves, and temperature in the twenties with light freezing spray.

S: This patient was found lying facedown on deck within seconds of being seen upright at the rail. The unsecured gear was clear of the scene and the patient's position was momentarily stable.

O: He was breathing and U on the AVPU scale for about two minutes before beginning to respond to questions. Once he was secure belowdecks, further exam showed swelling and discoloration on the back of his head, but no other injury. He complained of headache and vomited twice. Vital signs at 05:00: P: 60; R: 12; BP: 140/72; S: warm, dry; T: 97.0 rectally; C: V on AVPU.

A: Head injury (concussion)

A': 1. Elevated ICP

2. Airway obstruction from vomit

P: Secured in litter, wrapped to prevent heat loss. Fishing gear secured, Coast Guard notified, and the vessel underway for the nearest port. Airway constantly monitored.

Discussion: This is a nice neat case for evacuation. The patient's signs and symptoms fit the red flags for head injury. The patient was carefully monitored for signs of increasing ICP and any threat to the airway. The possibility of a helicopter evacuation was discussed with the Coast Guard, but the patient remained stable and did not vomit again. He arrived in port without incident.

Bones, Joints,

and Soft Tissue

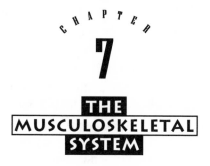

7

THE MUSCULOSKELETAL SYSTEM

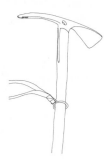

After giving the X rays one last look I noted my final diagnosis on the chart: "Mildly displaced fracture of the distal radius." What this really meant was "broken wrist," and the patient needed to see an orthopedic surgeon. Of course, she knew that when the accident happened, three days ago.

Karen was rock climbing above Chimney Pond on the north face of Maine's Mount Katahdin when a toehold pulled loose, dropping her six feet onto a small ledge. Her partner, Steve, immediately took up the slack in the rope and looked up to see if Karen needed further help.

She had landed on her right wrist and felt a crack and immediate pain, but a minute or two passed while Karen checked her position and equipment before she was able to assess her own injuries. Her wrist hurt, felt swollen, and her fingers were tingling. She had no other apparent injuries and her partner was able to lower her to the ground.

Steve conducted a patient survey and found that Karen was alert, fully oriented, and had no neck pain or tenderness. He noted the deformed and sore right wrist but continued his exam to be sure that it was the only injury. He used gentle traction to restore bone position, and a splint was fashioned using an aluminum stay from a backpack and a length of webbing for a sling. After a brief rest the two climbers hiked back to the cabin.

As Karen warmed up, the return of normal color and sensation to her fingers showed good blood perfusion beyond the injury. Even though she was pretty uncomfortable and sometimes light-headed and nauseated for the next several hours, Karen knew that this was no emergency.

There was no mechanism of injury that could cause volume shock. The feeling of faintness was part of a normal and harmless Acute Stress Reaction. The splint effectively stabilized the wrist, and elevation and cold compresses controlled the swelling and pain. Steve and Karen continued to monitor the fingers to ensure that circulation remained normal and were able to safely wait out the storm that closed in for the next two days.

These two climbers recognized that this wrist injury was more of a logistical dilemma than a medical emergency, even though they knew it was a fracture. Applying good common sense and basic understanding of the problem, they required neither rescue nor national news coverage.

Musculoskeletal injuries such as this are the most common backcountry medical problems. Although they are often a major inconvenience, they are rarely emergencies. Contrast Karen's story with one of my other favorites—the rescue of a teenaged girl in the mountains of Wyoming. During the traverse of a scree slope, a falling rock crushed the end of one of her fingers. She was in pain and scared and became anxious, light-headed, and pale. Even though there was no mechanism for severe volume loss, the trip leader decided that she was in "shock" and called for helicopter evacuation. The aircraft made an emergency flight in bad weather, and the patient was "saved." Although the rescue was very exciting and made a great story, the risk it created for the helicopter and crew was totally unjustified. This patient suffered only a crushed finger and Acute Stress Reaction.

You already know that life- or limb-threatening emergency involves a major problem with the neurological, respiratory, or circulatory system. It is extremely important to recognize these problems when they occur. But in the backcountry it can be just as important to recognize when they don't.

If you've taken a first-aid course you may recall a lot of concern over fractures of the femur (thigh bone), skull, spine, pelvis, and ribs. It is important to realize here that the real problems are not the fractured bones themselves but the potential injury to the vital organs next to them. Trauma patients do not die of fractures, sprains, strains, and contusions. They die from airway obstructions, blood loss, and brain injuries.

With a fractured femur or pelvis, we actually worry more about lacerated arteries (major circulatory system injury). With the ribs we are concerned with the lungs, liver, or spleen (circulatory and respiratory system). And with skull or spine fractures, it is the brain and spinal cord (neurological system) that's of real importance.

The important first step in handling any musculoskeletal problem is ruling out a major injury to one of the major body systems. Remember, your Initial Assessment should always focus on the vital functions of the respiratory, circulatory, and nervous systems, not broken bones or dislocated joints. Initially, suspected fractures in the pelvis, femur, spine, and skull should serve to focus your attention on the potential for major body system problems. If your Initial Assessment discovers no existing major injury, you have given yourself the luxury of time—time to perform a Focused History and Physical Exam, to think, treat, and safely evacuate yourself or your patient to medical care hours or days later. This may require help from rescue teams, but rarely as a hurried or risky undertaking.

STRUCTURE AND FUNCTION

Arms, legs, and fingers are moved by a system of cables, pulleys, and levers called tendons, ligaments, and bone. The motive power is

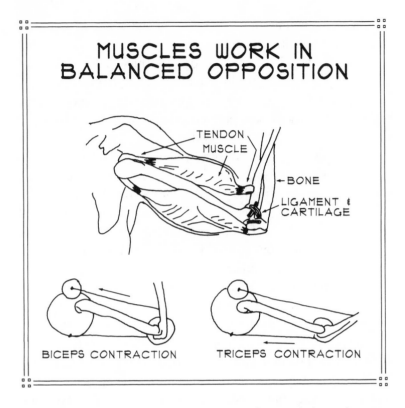

MUSCLES WORK IN BALANCED OPPOSITION

TENDON
MUSCLE
←BONE
LIGAMENT &
CARTILAGE

BICEPS CONTRACTION   TRICEPS CONTRACTION

supplied by the contraction of muscles working in balanced opposition across joints. The contraction of muscle on one side of the joint moves the bone one way, contraction on the other side moves it back.

Tendons are the tough connective tissue that join muscle to bone. Ligaments attach bone to bone across joints, and cartilage provides the smooth surfaces and padding on which bones slide against one another. There are, of course, many types of bones and joints but, knowing them in detail is not required for effective field treatment. A simple understanding of the basic system should help you get through any situation.

The spinal column with its stack of vertebrae is best viewed as another long bone with the head and pelvis as joints on either end. The same basic parts and principles are at work. The major difference is the complexity and importance of the adjacent soft tissue.

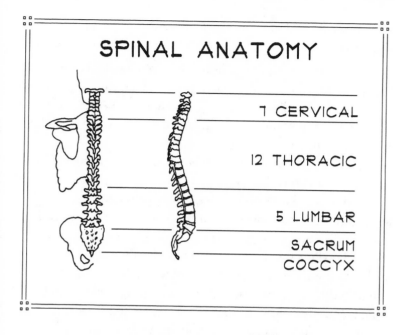

SPINAL ANATOMY

7 CERVICAL

12 THORACIC

5 LUMBAR

SACRUM

COCCYX

MUSCULOSKELETAL SYSTEM PROBLEMS

The familiar medical terminology used to describe musculoskeletal injury includes:

Contusions:	bruise of soft tissue or bone
Strains:	stretch injuries to muscle or tendon
Sprains:	stretch injuries to ligaments
Fractures:	broken bones or cartilage
Dislocations:	disruption of joints

More terms are added to indicate position and relative severity of injuries, for instance, describing a sprain as "grade 1" for a minor tear in a ligament, or "grade 3" for a complete rupture. Fractures can be comminuted, angulated, displaced, and further described with a dozen other interesting terms. But for field treatment in the back-country, the important distinction is simply whether the injury is *stable* or *unstable*.

UNSTABLE INJURIES: FRACTURES, DISLOCATIONS, AND SEVERE SPRAINS

Fractured bones and ruptured ligaments can result in unstable bone fragments and loose or displaced joints. This can cause severe damage to surrounding soft tissue such as muscles, nerves, and blood vessels. It is important to stabilize any injury in which fracture or ligament rupture is a possibility.

Fractures may be open (compound) or closed (simple). In an open fracture, the site is exposed to the outside environment through a wound in the skin. This opening can be produced from inside by sharp bone ends, or from outside by the same object that caused the fracture (like a bullet). Fortunately, open fractures are pretty rare.

A closed fracture is more difficult to diagnose because it is not visible to the naked eye. Because very few of us go into the backcountry with an X-ray machine, it is often impossible to tell if a bone is actually broken. In the field, when an injury has the mechanism, signs, and symptoms of instability, we treat it as such. Most fractures, severe sprains, and all dislocations fall into this category.

In talking about the assessment and treatment of unstable injuries, we will consider three main groups:

1. Extremity Fractures and severe sprains, requiring the stabilization of an individual extremity, such as an arm or ankle.

2. Dislocations, which may require manipulation or reduction (putting the dislocated bone back in place) as part of the stabilization.

3. Spine, pelvis, and femur fractures, requiring stabilization of the whole body.

EXTREMITY FRACTURES AND SEVERE SPRAINS

MECHANISM OF INJURY.

Fractures and sprains in extremities can be caused by a variety of mechanisms, reflecting the different ways force can be applied to bones and joints. The injury may be caused by leverage, twisting, direct impact, or a piece of bone being pulled away where the tendon or ligament attaches to it (avulsion fracture). For field purposes, however, defining mechanism of injury can be generalized to a yes or no question: Was there sufficient force to cause a fracture or rupture a ligament?

No doubt, almost everyone knows a person who broke a bone stepping off a curb or had a friend who limped around on "stress fractures" for weeks before being diagnosed. It's true, "sufficient force" can be difficult to define.

Positive Mechanism of Injury
Equals Sufficient Force for Unstable Injury

YES. A six-foot fall onto a ledge while rock climbing

NO. Waking up sore all over after a night sleeping on a ledge while rock climbing

---

ASSESSMENT OF EXTREMITY INJURY.

To the vague definition of sufficient force we add the not-so-vague signs and symptoms of instability. Combined with mechanism of injury, these provide a fairly clear guideline for identifying injuries that are likely to involve broken bones or other unstable elements, such as severe sprains.

Positive Mechanism Plus Positive Signs and Symptoms
Equals Unstable Injury

Positive Signs and Symptoms

The inability to move, use, or bear weight within a short time after injury.

The rapid onset of pain, tenderness, and swelling.

A history of feeling or hearing a snap, crack, or pop.

Obvious deformity or angulation.

The sensation of grating of bones against each other (crepitus) on movement.

The patient or examiner feels instability of bones or joints.

For example, consider two nearly identical swollen and sore knees on two nearly identically disgruntled skiers. Patient number one fell skiing early in the morning, twisting the knee. After resting for a few minutes, he was able to continue skiing well into the afternoon with only minor discomfort. The knee became sore and stiff after he stopped skiing for the day and soaked in a hot tub. It is now late evening, his knee is quite swollen, and he can barely move it.

Patient number two fell only thirty minutes ago, feeling a sharp pop and immediate pain. After the pain decreased a bit he tried to continue down the mountain, but the knee gave out, leaving him unable to control his skis. It is now quite swollen and immobile.

Both of these patients are grumpy and uncomfortable, and the pain prohibits a reliable examination of the knee, so it is the history that makes the difference in assessment. The first skier's story does not fit the description of an unstable injury. His severe discomfort twelve hours later is the result of the swelling and pressure in the joint that typically develops slowly after minor injury.

Patient number two, with the sharp pop and sense of instability clearly has an unstable injury. It is probably a ligament rupture and may or may not include a fracture. In any case, field treatment will require stabilization. His pain is due primarily to the rapid swelling from bleeding in the joint.

TREATMENT OF UNSTABLE EXTREMITY INJURY.

An extremity fracture or sprain by itself is never an emergency. As already mentioned, it is the potential for damage to the soft tissue around the injury site that is of real concern. The most important anticipated problem is extremity ischemia caused by lacerated or kinked blood vessels. Perfusion can also be lost when splints or bandages are tied too tightly, creating an artificial compartment syndrome. Treating the fracture or sprain correctly will fix or prevent this problem.

From the previous chapter, you know that nervous system tissue is the most sensitive to oxygen deprivation. With the onset of ischemia, peripheral nerves stop functioning and the extremity goes numb. With continued obstruction of perfusion, control of movement is lost as well.

The method of assessment for peripheral nerve function is checking circulation, sensation, and movement (CSM). You have experienced problems with CSM if you've slept on your arm or kept your backpack straps too tight. Circulation is impaired, the limb goes numb, and you can't move it. As circulation is restored movement returns, then tingling, then full sensation.

Circulation is checked by looking for evidence of blood flow in the injured extremity. Can you detect any pulses beyond (distal to) an area of injury? Is the skin normal in color, or pale, or blue? Is the skin colder than the same extremity on the other side?

Sensation is the most useful assessment tool. Loss of sensation is the first sign of ischemia. A normal limb will be able to feel the light touch of a finger or small object, an ischemic limb may not. In the early stages of ischemia, the patient may complain of a tingling sensation, then numbness. The loss of the ability to move the extremity, such as wiggling fingers or toes, develops later.

It is not unusual for an extremity to feel numb or cold immediately following injury, especially if the fracture results in deformity or the patient is having an Acute Stress Reaction. Your treatment will usually result in a significant improvement in CSM status as circulation is restored. Nevertheless, CSM may decay later, as swelling develops under a splint or wrap.

Extremity tissue can usually survive up to two hours of ischemia with minimal damage. Beyond this, the risk of tissue death and permanent damage increases quickly with time. *If your treatment efforts do not succeed in restoring CSM, you have a limb-threatening-emergency. Immediate evacuation is indicated if conditions permit.*

The generic treatment for unstable extremity injury has three distinct phases:

1. Traction into position
2. Hand stable
3. Splint stable

1. Traction into position (TIP). Injured bones and joints, and the soft tissues around them, are much more comfortable and much less likely to be damaged further if they are splinted in normal anatomic position. Although many injured extremities will remain in good position or return there on their own, some will require help from you.

To restore anatomic position of a fractured bone we first apply traction. Traction separates the bone ends and reduces pain. Then, while traction is maintained, position is restored. To understand how this works, picture moving a chain as a unit by keeping the links under tension rather than allowing them to rattle against one another.

Shaft fractures of long bones are brought into the line of normal bone axis, the "in-line" position. This is where the effect of opposing muscles is most balanced and the blood circulation to the extremity beyond the injury is best maintained. If you're not sure what the realigned extremity should look like, check the opposite extremity. That's why people have two of almost everything.

Injured joints, such as elbows, shoulders, and knees, usually do not need to be repositioned. If your patient is conscious and mobile he will have already found the most comfortable position for the injured joint and will be holding it there by the time you come along. If not, applying gentle TIP to a position in the midrange of the joint's normal motion is the best approach for long-term care.

In severely deformed joints, such as dislocations, there is likely to be a loss of circulation, sensation, and movement (CSM) beyond the injury site. Under these conditions, TIP with movement toward the midrange position is used until circulation is reestablished. In some specific cases that we'll discuss later, TIP can be used to reduce dislocations (put the dislocated bone back in place) and significantly improve the patient's comfort and circulation.

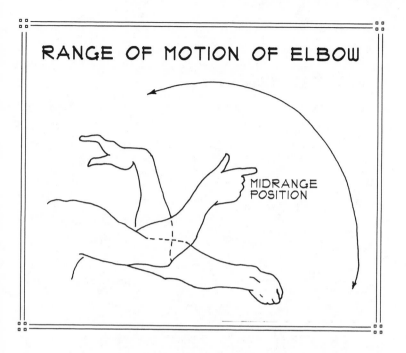

RANGE OF MOTION OF ELBOW

MIDRANGE
POSITION

Traction into position is a safe procedure if done properly. It generally decreases pain rather than increases it. However, to be successful it helps to have the cooperation and confidence of the injured person. Pulling on a fractured leg without telling its owner how or why you're going to do it won't win you any friends. If necessary, you and your assistants may want to practice on an uninjured limb first.

Occasionally it will be impossible to comfortably and safely restore position, even using TIP. You should discontinue TIP and stabilize the injury in the position it was found if TIP causes a significant increase in pain or if movement of the extremity is prevented by resistance.

Open-shaft fractures with bone ends protruding through the skin are still managed with TIP. Bone ends often move back beneath the skin surface when traction is applied, so it is best to first clean the exposed bone by irrigating it with water and brushing away debris (see the section in Chapter 8 on high-risk wounds). Clean the surrounding skin with antiseptic solution or soap and water. Try to keep the skin of the wound edges from becoming trapped under the bone as you realign the fracture. You may have to pull it free with a clean tweezers or a gloved finger as the bone is manipulated back into the wound.

Hand Stable. Once you have repositioned an extremity injury, stability must be maintained until the splint can take over. This may mean having someone maintain gentle traction on the extremity while you collect materials. If you don't have an army of assistants you may have to use snow, rocks, or pieces of equipment to hold the limb in place. Don't just drop it without some kind of support. Of course, if you were really thinking, you might have had your splint materials ready before you started the process.

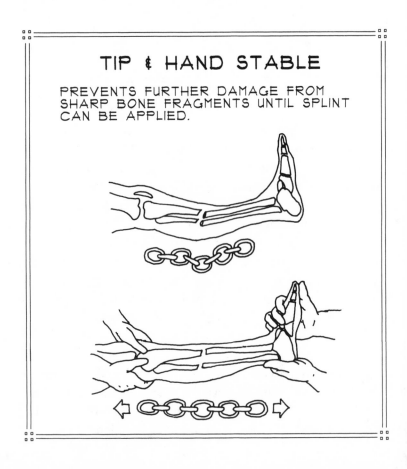

TIP ¢ HAND STABLE

PREVENTS FURTHER DAMAGE FROM SHARP BONE FRAGMENTS UNTIL SPLINT CAN BE APPLIED.

Splint Stable. Splinting is a real art in first aid. We've seen an incredible variety of splints, from fabulously expensive stainless steel jobs with dozens of moving parts to disorganized collections of firewood and baling twine. The best of them are simple, light, cheap, and probably in your backpack or boat right now. The most useful splinting materials include sleeping pads, backpack stays, snowshoes, flotation vests, nylon webbing, and giant safety pins.

What—you don't carry giant safety pins? You should. This marvelous device (also known as a diaper pin) weighs practically nothing, takes up no space, and costs only a few cents, yet it can convert a shirt or jacket into an instant sling and swathe for wrist, arm, and shoulder injuries. It is almost as useful as duct tape, the other item you should never leave home without.

Duct tape is that silver stuff, very sticky and strong, that is nevertheless easy to tear into pieces with your hands. It can be warmed

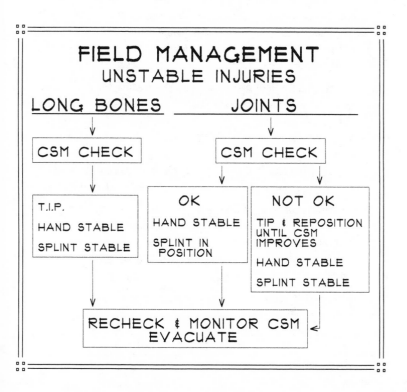

FIELD MANAGEMENT
UNSTABLE INJURIES

LONG BONES _____ JOINTS

CSM CHECK ___ CSM CHECK

T.I.P.
HAND STABLE
SPLINT STABLE

OK
HAND STABLE
SPLINT IN POSITION

NOT OK
TIP & REPOSITION UNTIL CSM IMPROVES
HAND STABLE
SPLINT STABLE

RECHECK & MONITOR CSM
EVACUATE

with a lighter in cold and wet weather and will stick to almost any surface. With a few yards of duct tape and that giant safety pin, you can splint or fix just about everything.

In addition, there is one commercial splint material worthy of mention. It is call a SAM Splint and consists of a strip of malleable aluminum sandwiched between layers of foam padding. It can be bent and cut to create a variety of lightweight but strong splints for the wrist, ankle, and fingers. It can even be made into a reasonable cervical collar for neck injuries.

Principles of Splinting.

Regardless of how you make it, an improvised splint should be complete, comfortable, and compact. Be sure to pay attention to all three qualities. Duct-taping someone's arm to a canoe would do a fine job of immobilizing the wrist but wouldn't be very comfortable, and the evacuation would be dangerous, to say the least. Splints should be:

1. Complete. Splint in the in-line position, including the joint above and below the injury. For example, to effectively splint a lower-leg fracture, the ankle and knee must be immobilized. Joint injuries are splinted in the midrange position, including the bones above and below the injury. For example, to splint the elbow, include the forearm and upper arm in the splint. There is no need to include adjacent joints in the splint—the shoulder and wrist may be left mobile.

2. Comfortable. A splint should be well padded, strong, and snug. There should be no movement of the injured bones, and no pressure points or loose spots. Your splint should improve and preserve blood perfusion and nerve function, not impair it. A good splint will result in decreased pain and intact CSM.

3. Compact. A splint should be no larger or more complex than necessary. It should allow you to monitor distal CSM and loosen or adjust the splint if ischemia develops. It should not inhibit evacuation.

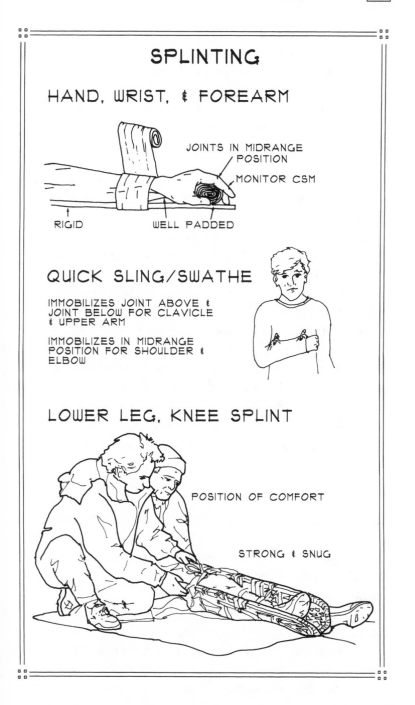

SPLINTING

HAND, WRIST, & FOREARM

JOINTS IN MIDRANGE
POSITION

MONITOR CSM

RIGID   WELL PADDED

QUICK SLING/SWATHE

IMMOBILIZES JOINT ABOVE &
JOINT BELOW FOR CLAVICLE
& UPPER ARM

IMMOBILIZES IN MIDRANGE
POSITION FOR SHOULDER &
ELBOW

LOWER LEG, KNEE SPLINT

POSITION OF COMFORT

STRONG & SNUG

Once the extremity is stabilized with your perfect splint and you are satisfied that CSM is improving, treatment should include rest and elevation to reduce swelling and pressure (see the section on treatment of stable injuries later in this chapter). As long as distal CSM remains normal or continues to improve, you can take your time planning a safe and comfortable evacuation.

JOINT DISLOCATIONS

The average garden variety joint is a complex mobile assembly of bones, ligaments, cartilage, tendon, and muscle. To the delight of orthopedic surgeons everywhere, these structures can be injured in a wide variety of combinations and levels of severity. A dislocation occurs when enough force is applied to the bone to tear the restraining ligaments and allow the joint to come apart.

By definition, dislocations have mechanisms of injury, signs, and symptoms of unstable injuries, and we treat them by the same general principles. Stabilize the joint in the midrange position and evacuate to treatment. There are, however, three specific dislocations that deserve special attention because they are easy and safe to fix in the field: simple dislocations of the shoulder, patella (kneecap), and digits (fingers and toes). This can save a lot of pain and trouble and will make you into a real hero by transforming a gruesome medical emergency into a minor logistical problem.

SHOULDER DISLOCATIONS

MECHANISM OF INJURY.

Simple dislocations are caused by *indirect injury*, where force is applied at a distance from the joint and the dislocation is caused by leverage or torque. The usual mechanism is forced external rotation. Fractures are uncommon with shoulder dislocation and generally do not interfere with treatment.

These injuries can be extremely uncomfortable and result in significant ischemia to the joint and surrounding soft tissue, with damage increasing significantly after a couple of hours. The benefit of early reduction, even by an inexperienced rescuer, generally outweighs the risk of causing further damage with manipulation.

Reduction is best accomplished within an hour of the injury, before severe swelling and muscle spasm develops.

The more serious dislocation, from *direct injury*, is usually the result of high-speed impact into a solid object. Because sufficient force is applied directly to the joint area to force the bone ends apart, distinguishing this from indirect force is usually not difficult. These injuries are almost always associated with other major trauma.

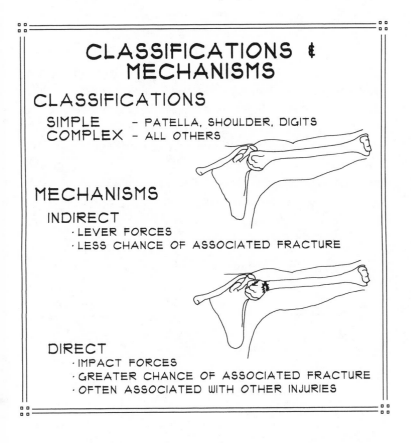

CLASSIFICATIONS & MECHANISMS

CLASSIFICATIONS

SIMPLE — PATELLA, SHOULDER, DIGITS
COMPLEX — ALL OTHERS

MECHANISMS

INDIRECT
· LEVER FORCES
· LESS CHANCE OF ASSOCIATED FRACTURE

DIRECT
· IMPACT FORCES
· GREATER CHANCE OF ASSOCIATED FRACTURE
· OFTEN ASSOCIATED WITH OTHER INJURIES

ASSESSMENT OF SHOULDER DISLOCATION.

When you are trying to determine if a simple dislocation can be fixed in the field, it is important to pay careful attention to the mechanism of injury during your surveys and history.

You can be relatively sure that you are dealing with a simple dislocation if the patient describes the classic mechanism of forced external rotation, such as overextending the arm while trying to brake a skiing fall or high bracing with a kayak paddle. In many cases, there is a history of recurrent dislocation in the same extremity. You'll notice right away that the person with a dislocated shoulder is in moderate to severe discomfort. Acute Stress Reaction is common. In about half the cases there is some CSM impairment of the arm and hand. The shoulder itself loses the rounded contour and becomes a "step-off deformity," with a hollow area where the shoulder is normally full and rounded. It is likely that the patient will be unwilling to move the shoulder joint without help and coaching.

Occasionally a shoulder dislocation can be confused with a shoulder separation, which is a disruption of the joint between the distal end of the clavicle and the scapula (Acromioclavicular joint). The usual mechanism of injury is a direct blow to the top of the shoulder during a fall. This joint lies directly above the shoulder joint and can have a step-off appearance when injured. The key difference is that, in separation, the shoulder joint and upper arm remain mobile. In dislocation, mobility is lost.

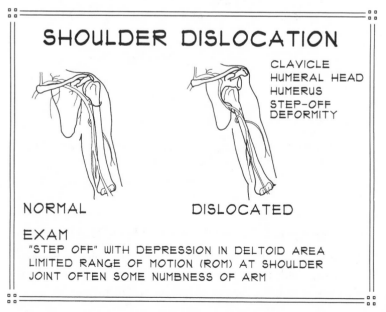

SHOULDER DISLOCATION

NORMAL   DISLOCATED

CLAVICLE
HUMERAL HEAD
HUMERUS
STEP-OFF
DEFORMITY

EXAM
"STEP OFF" WITH DEPRESSION IN DELTOID AREA
LIMITED RANGE OF MOTION (ROM) AT SHOULDER
JOINT OFTEN SOME NUMBNESS OF ARM

TREATMENT OF SHOULDER DISLOCATION.

A simple dislocation of the shoulder should be reduced in the field if the evacuation time to definitive care will be greater than two hours. It should also be considered if the evacuation will be exceptionally difficult or dangerous to perform while the shoulder remains displaced. These criteria apply to most backcountry and marine situations.

There are a number of techniques that are effective in reducing dislocated shoulders, but the best we've found for field use requires only a small patch of level ground and one rescuer. Because it is performed gently and slowly, it carries a low risk of causing further injury.

To begin, the patient's arm is supported while the patient is moved to a position lying on his back. Gentle traction on the upper arm will help relieve pain during movement. The patient's cooperation and relaxation is essential. Take your time—there is no reason to torture your patient with speed. Once the patient is lying on his back, the rescuer applies gentle traction to the arm and slowly swings it into a position about 90 degrees from the body, with the elbow bent.

The rescuer continues to maintain TIP with one hand just above the elbow. Traction should be firm, but not enough to slide the patient across the ground. There should be no need for countertraction. The patient should be gently and repeatedly encouraged to relax his shoulder muscles.

With the other hand on the patient's forearm, the rescuer gently and slowly externally rotates the arm until the "baseball position" is reached. This looks just like it sounds: It is exactly the position the patient would have his arm in if he were throwing a ball. Once the arm is in this position, make yourself comfortable and continue gentle traction. Frequently remind your patient to relax his shoulder muscles. Tell him that he must let the joint return to its normal position with the muscles in balance.

Usually, within five to ten minutes, the muscles will fatigue, allowing the joint to slip back into place. If nothing has happened after about fifteen minutes, try a move called "throwing the baseball." Again, this looks exactly like it sounds. Watch the patient's shoulder and pick a moment when you see the muscles really relax.

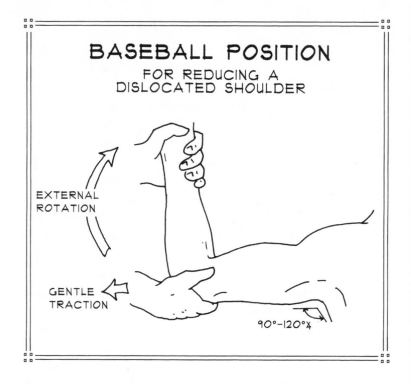

BASEBALL POSITION
FOR REDUCING A
DISLOCATED SHOULDER

EXTERNAL
ROTATION

GENTLE
TRACTION

90°–120°

Gently rotate the arm and hand forward as if the patient were throwing a ball. This is almost always successful in encouraging the shoulder to pop back into its socket.

You will know when the shoulder joint has been reduced by a dramatic relief of pain and the return of mobility to the joint. You can often feel and see a sudden shift of the upper arm as it relocates in the socket. If CSM impairment was present before reduction, it will rapidly improve afterward. Remember to check and document CSM both before and after reduction.

Following reduction, your patient usually experiences significant relief and will thank you profusely enough to embarrass you. Enjoy it, but remember that a joint dislocation has the positive mechanism, signs, and symptoms of an unstable injury. Inevitably, swelling and pressure will develop and pain will increase over time. The most effective splint for this is a simple sling. The patient should plan for medical follow-up within a week, if possible.

Some shoulders will remain quite painful immediately after reduction. This is especially true of dislocations in which a small piece of bone has been chipped off of the ball of the humerus. As long as distal circulation and sensation (CSM) is intact, however, this should not be a cause for alarm. Nevertheless, an early medical follow-up is a good idea.

Dislocations that result from direct force are generally more complicated and usually not reduced in the field. Manipulation is directed only at restoring CSM, if necessary, and at positioning the patient for safe evacuation. If the patient is to be walked out, a sling pinned to the patient's shirt or jacket is effective immobilization.

PATELLA DISLOCATION

MECHANISM OF INJURY.

The patella (kneecap) is an isolated bone imbedded as a kind of fulcrum in the quadriceps tendon. This large tendon transmits the powerful force of the quadriceps muscle in the front of the thigh to the front of the lower leg, allowing extension of the knee. This is the motion you'd use to bring your foot forward, kick a ball, or kick your climbing partner for dropping you.

The quadriceps tendon passes over and through a groove in the femur like a cable running through a pulley. In patellar dislocation the cable, with the patella included, slips off the femur, making it impossible for the knee to function.

Like the shoulder, the patella can dislocate with a direct blow (this is rare) or indirect mechanism, typically a sudden extension of the knee while twisting or turning. The patient often has a history of recurrent dislocation. The dislocation is always lateral (to the outside), leaving the patella pinned against the outside of the knee by the pull of the quadriceps.

ASSESSMENT OF PATELLA DISLOCATION.

The appearance of a dislocated kneecap can be deceiving. Shifting the patella laterally will make the bony prominence on the inside of the knee stand out and look like the missing patella. Don't be fooled. Feel for the patella laterally—you'll find it.

As with the shoulder, these dislocations are extremely uncomfortable, and there is little or no motion of the joint. Distal circulation and sensation is usually unaffected, but you should check it anyway. Damage to surrounding soft tissue will increase with time, as will the difficulty of reduction.

TREATMENT OF PATELLA DISLOCATION.

A dislocated patella should be reduced if the evacuation time will be greater than two hours or if the evacuation will be unreasonably difficult. Reducing a dislocated patella is also reversing the mechanism of injury. Take the tension off the "cable" by flexing the hip (have the patient sit up). Then straighten the knee. If the patella does not relocate on its own, a gentle push with your thumbs will usually do the trick. As with the shoulder, relief of pain and return of mobility will indicate success. Also like the shoulder, these injuries are likely to result in swelling and significant pain later.

Ideally, a reduced patella dislocation should be splinted as an unstable injury and the patient carried out. However, in less than ideal situations the knee could be braced and the patient walked out if pain permits. As with the shoulder, the key is to avoid repeating the mechanism of injury. As long as CSM is OK, there is no emergency. As always, however, medical follow-up is important.

DIGIT DISLOCATIONS—FINGERS AND TOES

MECHANISM OF INJURY.

Joints in the fingers usually dislocate due to an indirect force that levers the bone ends apart. The classic example is catching a falling softball the wrong way. Instead of dropping neatly in the palm of your hand, the ball hits the tips of your fingers, levering the bones backward, and dislocating a joint. You easily can do the same thing catching a falling climber or a drifting canoe. In any case, what you end up with is a finger pointing the wrong way at the distal or middle joint.

These dislocations often have an associated small chip fracture. Motion of the dislocated joint is impossible, and there will be some degree of CSM impairment. As with all dislocations, damage from ischemia will increase with time.

TREATMENT OF DIGIT DISLOCATION.

Your first reaction when confronted with a dislocated finger will be to want to put it back where it belongs, especially if it is yours. Fortunately, this is exactly what should be done if definitive care will be delayed more than two hours. TIP for this type of dislocation is the same as for shaft fractures. Reduction will be most easily accomplished right after the injury has occurred, before the swelling and pain get worse.

After getting your patient's consent, simply grasp the end of the offending finger with one hand and the rest of the finger in the other. Slowly but firmly pull the end of the finger first in the direction it is pointing, then, while maintaining traction, swing it back in line. This is not as easy as it sounds, but it does work. You'll probably need to wrap the end of your patient's finger in gauze or a bandanna to help assure your grip.

After reduction, resist the temptation to play with the finger. You should, however, place a splint in the midrange of the joint's motion because fracture is very likely and the finger will need medical attention. Also, remember to check CSM before and after reduction. Things should improve with your treatment.

DIFFICULT DISLOCATIONS

In the backcountry any dislocation that resists your efforts at reduction can become a serious problem. Pain may be severe, and the potential for tissue damage due to ischemia increases with time. If CSM is significantly impaired and cannot be restored by traction and repositioning, immediate evacuation to medical care is warranted. These are limb-threatening emergencies.

SPINE, FEMUR, AND PELVIS FRACTURES

In stabilizing musculoskeletal injuries to the spine, pelvis, and femur, we apply the same assessment skills and splinting principles as in extremity injury. Effective splinting of these bones usually requires a long backboard, vacuum splint, or litter that can secure the hips, back, and neck. Needless to say, this pretty well eliminates walking your patient out of the woods in all but the most desperate situations. The equipment necessary is brought to the scene by rescue teams or aircraft and requires a carry-out or airlift evacuation. While you are waiting, you will need to shelter and stabilize the patient in place or move her to shelter in a safe location.

S P I N E   F R A C T U R E

M E C H A N I S M   O F   I N J U R Y .

The spine is fractured like any other bone, by both direct and indirect trauma. All spine injury is significant, but the most potentially devastating is the fracture or dislocation of the cervical spine (neck).

The delicate tissue of the spinal cord, really an extension of the brain, is surrounded and protected by the bones of the spinal column. Unstable injuries of the bony spinal column can easily injure the cord. Cord injury above the level of the third vertebra in the neck will cause respiratory arrest. Below that level, injuries usually result in quadriplegia, that is, loss of function in all four extremities. These injuries are usually permanent, but recovery is sometimes possible with careful treatment.

The neck is the most commonly injured area because it is the most mobile section of the spine, linking the heavy mass of the head with the body. As a result, it is very prone to injury whenever the head is snapped back and forth like a ball on a string. It is also subject to damage when a force is applied to the top of the head, for instance, being struck by a rockfall, or diving into shallow water and striking bottom. There is a logical association between head injury and neck fracture. *In the presence of head injury, cervical spine injury is always assumed to exist until proven otherwise!*

Injury to the spine at the thoracic (chest) level is much less common, because the added rigidity of the rib cage makes this the most stable area of the spine. It also means that injury at this level is likely to be associated with other major chest trauma from significant force. Spinal cord injury in the thorax can cause paraplegia or loss of function of the lower extremities.

Below the thorax is the lumbar spine which, like the neck, is less protected and more mobile. Unstable injuries are more common here, but cord injury is rare. Near the top of the lumbar spine the spinal cord separates into individual nerve roots that look like a loose bundle of linguine. These nerve roots are mobile and less likely than the spinal cord to be injured directly.

Assessment of Spine Fracture.

The signs and symptoms of spine fracture are really no different than those of other fractures, but because the consequences of spinal cord injury are so devastating, we tend to be much more conservative in our assessment and treatment. On the street, ambulance crews routinely immobilize any trauma patient with a positive mechanism for spine injury. This makes sense in situations where the patient will arrive at the hospital within a few minutes and a full assessment can be made in the more controlled environment of the emergency department.

In the backcountry or far out to sea, however, we realize that committing a patient and rescuers to full spinal immobilization and evacuation can be impractical and even dangerous. We cannot afford to transport everyone who takes a tumble in the woods out on a backboard. Our field assessment must be able to "clear" some patients of spine injury, even in the presence of a positive mechanism.

When we examine a patient who has sustained enough trauma to cause spine injury, we look for the same signs and symptoms of unstable injury used in extremity trauma. But because the spinal cord may be involved, we must consider the possibility that normal body reactions, such as feeling pain, may be absent. This is especially true when spinal injury is accompanied by head injury or ASR. A critical part of your assessment has to do with the reliability of your own exam.

When your patient's consciousness and mental status is altered due to head injury, intoxication, or Acute Stress Reaction, your examination will be unreliable. In this case, it is best to assume that a positive mechanism means spine injury—no matter what your exam shows—and treat it as such. You can evaluate again later when your patient may have cleared her head, calmed down, or sobered up. In the backcountry this could happen before you leave camp to get help, or at any time during the evacuation.

If your patient is or becomes calm, cooperative, sober, and alert, your examination can be considered reliable. To "clear" the spine from suspicion of injury, there should be no complaint of spine pain, no tenderness as you examine the length of the spine with your fingers, and no complaint of numbness or tingling of extremities. The patient should be able to demonstrate good muscle function (also called motor function) by holding her fingers open against resistance, and by pushing her toes and wrists up and down firmly and equally. The patient should be able to feel the difference between a sharp object and a soft touch on both hands and feet. If the patient passes all of these tests there is no spine injury, and there is no need for spinal immobilization. Performing this type of exam may seem

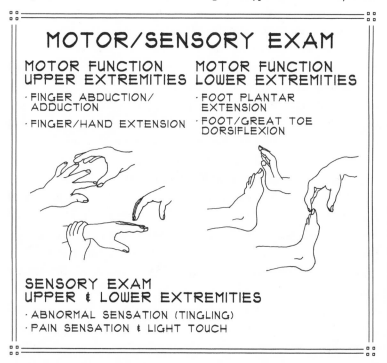

MOTOR/SENSORY EXAM

MOTOR FUNCTION UPPER EXTREMITIES

· FINGER ABDUCTION/ ADDUCTION
· FINGER/HAND EXTENSION

MOTOR FUNCTION LOWER EXTREMITIES

· FOOT PLANTAR EXTENSION
· FOOT/GREAT TOE DORSIFLEXION

SENSORY EXAM UPPER & LOWER EXTREMITIES

· ABNORMAL SENSATION (TINGLING)
· PAIN SENSATION & LIGHT TOUCH

like a lot of work at the time, but clearing the spine as a cause for concern will vastly simplify your problem list.

Any positive findings during the exam, such as tenderness or the inability to move extremities equally, means that you should treat for spine injury. Later examination on the evacuation route or in the hospital may clear the spine but for now you are obligated to stabilize the spine as best you can under the circumstances.

It is important to note that many patients who have been involved in accidents on the highway, rocks, or ski slopes develop lots of minor aches and pains as swelling and inflammation increase over

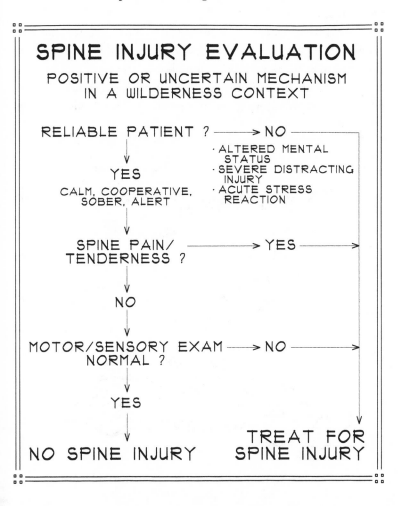

SPINE INJURY EVALUATION

POSITIVE OR UNCERTAIN MECHANISM
IN A WILDERNESS CONTEXT

RELIABLE PATIENT ? ———→ NO ———
            ↓   · ALTERED MENTAL
           YES   STATUS
                                 · SEVERE DISTRACTING
   CALM, COOPERATIVE,   INJURY
     SOBER, ALERT   · ACUTE STRESS
                                   REACTION

            ↓
     SPINE PAIN/ ———————→ YES ————————→
   TENDERNESS ?

            ↓
           NO

            ↓
MOTOR/SENSORY EXAM ——→ NO ————————→
     NORMAL ?

            ↓
           YES

            ↓   ↓
                              TREAT FOR
NO SPINE INJURY   SPINE INJURY

several hours. A stiff neck is one of these common late-occurring symptoms. As long as you were able to clear the spine initially and have not dropped your patient on her head since, this new onset of pain does not warrant immobilization.

TREATMENT OF SPINE FRACTURE.

For field purposes, the spine is treated as a long bone with a joint at each end. The positioning and treatment principles are the same as for a long-bone fracture. The techniques will vary depending on the equipment available, the terrain to be crossed, and the people providing first aid.

Use TIP to restore the injured spine to the normal anatomic position (head level, eyes ahead, and the shoulders and pelvis in the same plane). As with other long bones, the spine will be most stable and least likely to injure adjacent nerves and blood vessels when it is in this normal in-line position. This is also best for airway protection.

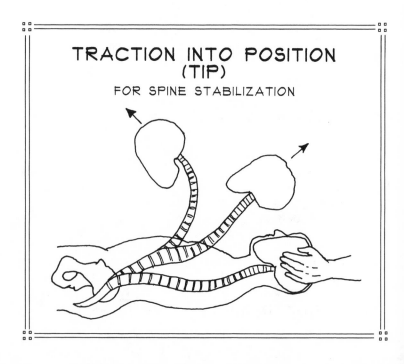

TRACTION INTO POSITION (TIP)

FOR SPINE STABILIZATION

Use hand stable to maintain the normal alignment of the spine throughout any lifting, rolling, or carrying. The next step is splint stable, which secures the head and neck by a collar, and immobilizes the lower spine and pelvis with a long board or litter. Although splinting is best accomplished with equipment designed for this purpose, you can improvise and make very effective splints and collars from camping equipment.

In most cases where you cannot clear the spine, you will be better off setting up camp right where you are and sending a runner for help. While you're waiting, lay your patient on a pad and sleeping bag for comfort and insulation. You can block the head with packs or clothing to prevent movement. The patient will need help with everything, including eating, drinking, urinating, and defecating. Because your patient will be unable to exercise to generate body heat, you must be careful to keep her well fed, hydrated, warm, and dry.

If waiting for rescue is not an option, you should provide the maximum stability possible to the patient's spine before movement. Carrying the patient supine in an improvised litter with a cervical collar in place is best (a very effective custom-made collar can be cut from an Ensolite pad or made with a SAM Splint). There are times, however, when the benefits of immobilizing the patient are outweighed by the risks of a carry-out evacuation. There might be no other option in some circumstances but to have a person walk or climb with a potential spine injury. Though it is occasionally necessary, it should be the absolute last resort.

FEMUR FRACTURE

The femur (long bone in the thigh) is part of the lower extremity and structurally is similar to the other long bones in the leg and arm, though much bigger. It is not easy to fracture a femur—to do so requires massive force. We group femur fracture with spine and pelvis injuries because, unlike the other extremities, these require whole-body stabilization. The hip and pelvis form the joint above the injury, requiring a litter or backboard to secure. The added stability also helps prevent additional damage from the powerful thigh muscles, which are easily thrown into spasm by movement.

ASSESSMENT OF FEMUR FRACTURE.

Of the signs and symptoms of fracture, the one most typical of femur fracture is severe pain. Unless there is pain masking from another injury or intoxication, the patient will be extremely uncomfortable. Movement is difficult, and bearing weight is impossible.

A suspected femur fracture should make you think of the possibility of volume shock from major circulatory system injury. The large femoral artery runs close to the bone and can be lacerated by broken bone ends. Even in a closed fracture of the femur, considerable blood can be lost into the thigh. The original problem may be a fractured femur, but the more serious anticipated problem is volume shock.

TREATMENT OF FEMUR FRACTURE.

Firm TIP reduces pain and spasm, reduces the chance of injury to arteries and nerves, and reduces the space available inside the thigh for blood loss. TIP should be applied as soon as possible whenever femur fracture is recognized, and it should be maintained through the splinting process.

The ideal femur splint would maintain traction all the way to the hospital, and there are several types of specialized traction splints made for this purpose. These splints require training and experience to use and even when properly applied can impair circulation. This quickly becomes a problem in a long-term-care situation and requires careful monitoring.

Improvised traction splints for field use employing ski poles, canoe paddles, and other pieces of equipment are often more architecturally interesting than medically useful. If you think you may have to use one of these, test your idea and work out the details before you subject your patient to it. If you're not so sure of your design, remember that firm immobilization on a long board or litter is simple, safe, and effective.

PELVIC FRACTURE
MECHANISM OF INJURY.

As with the femur, it takes significant force to fracture the pelvis. Pelvic injuries are usually associated with long falls, high-speed ski accidents, and avalanches. As with the femur, a major concern is the possibility of severe bleeding from arteries and veins adjacent to the fracture site.

ASSESSMENT OF PELVIC FRACTURE.

Pelvic fractures have no single outstanding signs or symptoms, making them a tricky injury to diagnose. They are usually quite painful, but not always. They can also be difficult to distinguish from hip or lower lumbar spine fractures. In the presence of positive mechanism, pelvic pain and tenderness, and inability to bear weight, you have little choice but to treat for fracture.

TREATMENT OF PELVIC FRACTURE.

Pelvic fracture requires immobilization of the trunk to meet the principles of splinting. Because of danger to adjacent blood vessels, possible pelvic fractures deserve long-board or litter stabilization also. Volume shock should be in your anticipated problem list if it's not already present. As with femur fracture, it is often going to be best to stabilize the patient in place and call for help with evacuation.

STABLE INJURIES

Nearly every morning, even before the lifts have opened, there are a couple of skiers waiting for the clinic to open. Anyone in ski-area medicine will recognize them—one leg stiff, furrowed brow, frown on the face. This is the stable knee injury.

Paul had been skiing the snowfield above King Pine chair yesterday when he caught a ski tip on a tree and twisted the lower leg outward. He felt mild pain in the right knee but was able to continue skiing for several more hours.

He felt no pop or snap at the time of injury, and no instability afterward. It was not until later in the evening that the pain and swelling began. He soaked in the hot tub for an hour and went to bed.

Today Paul's knee is very sore. There is slight swelling and tenderness on the inside of the joint. There is good range of motion, but with considerable pain. Even with these findings today, the history indicates that Paul has a stable injury.

The treatment for Paul's injury is rest, ice, elevation, and compression (RICE). During the first forty-eight hours after injury heat should not be applied because it will just increase the swelling. After a day or so Paul can return to whatever activity is possible without causing significant pain (pain-free activity). He should be ready to ski again in a few days or weeks.

ASSESSMENT OF STABLE INJURIES.

Typical signs and symptoms of stable injury include positive mechanism and pain, but none of the specific signs and symptoms of fracture. The patient is able to use or move the limb or bear weight within the first hour following injury. There is no history of a snap, crack, or pop. There is no deformity, crepitus, or sense of instability.

Swelling is common, but it develops slowly over several hours from the development of edema rather than rapidly from bleeding. It is not unusual for the patient to experience considerable pain and immobility the day after the injury as this swelling and pressure reach a peak. This is especially true if the patient continued to use the injured part for a while after the injury.

TREATMENT OF STABLE INJURIES.

The ideal early treatment of stable injuries is essentially the same as that for unstable ones. This conservative treatment prevents the development of disability from excessive pain and swelling during the first twenty-four hours. The handy acronym is

> **RICE**
> **Rest.** Local rest means splinted or limited use.
> **Ice.** Use as tolerated during first twenty-four hours.
> **Compression.** Use an Ace Bandage only on distal extremity.
> **Elevation.** Raise the injury above heart level.

PAIN-FREE ACTIVITY (PFA).

After the first twenty-four hours, or when most of the pain and swelling has resolved, the injured person may resume activity as long as additional pain is not caused. This may include skiing, or it may require very limited movement around camp for several days.

MEDICATION.

Anti-inflammatory medication such as aspirin or ibuprofen can help reduce swelling and discomfort. Using them regularly for several days to raise the level of the drug in the body works better than just taking them occasionally in response to pain.

Remember the six- to twenty-four-hour swelling curve? Elevation and rest are the most important elements of RICE and are most useful early on, while the swelling is likely to be worst. Ice is also very helpful. Even in the summer you can achieve some evaporative cooling by wrapping the injury in a water-soaked bandage.

Under these treatment guidelines, all stable injuries should show steady improvement. If not, your patient is being too active, or your assessment may be wrong. It *is* possible to have a stable injury with a small fracture, which causes prolonged discomfort. Never be afraid to reassess the situation and change your mind. Medical people do it all the time.

TENDINITIS

This is a good time to talk about the meaning of the suffix *itis*. It is a nonspecific term indicating inflammation or irritation. Tendinitis is inflammation of a tendon, arthritis is inflammation of a joint, appendicitis is inflammation of the appendix. The term does not specify *why* the part is inflamed. The cause may be infection, trauma, sunburn, anything capable of causing damage. "Itis" is really a symptom of a more specific problem.

In the case of tendons, muscles, ligaments, and cartilage, the usual cause of inflammation in wilderness travel is overuse, or repetitive motion injury. Anything subject to repeated friction will wear out eventually—ropes, sails, boot soles, your favorite toothbrush. Your body parts are no exception. What is exceptional about your body is its ability to repair the damage if you can give it enough time.

Assessment of Tendinitis.

Tendinitis, such as the kind that develops in a kayaker's wrist, is a symptom of too much wear and too little time for repair. You will note the typical pain, swelling, and sometimes redness over the inflamed muscle and tendon structure. Moving it will hurt, and you may be able to feel crepitus as the damaged tendon slides roughly through the irritated tendon sheath. Resting the muscles and tendons will feel better.

These symptoms are typical of all kinds of repetitive motion injury. Bikers get it in the knee, hikers in the foot, rowers in the wrists, and writers in the hands. The field treatment is pretty much the same for all.

Treatment of Tendinitis.

You have to break the cycle of injury and inflammation. That is, stop doing what hurts. This is easy to say but difficult to do. If possible, splint the limb to minimize the motion of the part that hurts. As pain subsides, remove the splint two or three times a day and do gentle exercises, taking the injured part through its normal range of motion as pain allows.

Take anti-inflammatory medication like ibuprofen over several days. After the initial inflammation has settled down, apply heat, using warm soaks four times a day for fifteen minutes at a time. This is good to do just before the range-of-motion exercises.

And how do these fine suggestions help you on day five of a week-and-a-half river trip? Unfortunately, the cause, problem, and symptoms of tendinitis remain the same. You will have to address the treatment differently in order to keep moving.

You might try to change the way you perform the repetitive motion, putting the stress on different muscle-and-tendon groups. For example, using a short loop of webbing as a handle on a kayak paddle can allow you to pull it with your wrist held vertically instead of horizontally. You won't have the control you're used to, but it may keep you moving.

Take the full therapeutic dose of anti-inflammatory medication. For ibuprofen this is 3,200 milligrams a day. Your stomach may allow a couple of days of this, which may suppress the inflammation enough to prevent complete disability.

Using tape and padding, you can create a soft splint that will help reduce the stress on the irritated structure. Joint taping is a science in itself and beyond the scope of this book, but it's worth learning if you are responsible for kayak, canoe, and hiking groups. Rest frequently. Let pain be your guide. Stop immediately when the pain begins to grow worse. Continue only after it is under control.

Case Study—Musculoskeletal System

S: A twenty-three-year-old female instructor glissading a snow-field in the Tetons caught her heel in the snow, causing a tumbling fall. She felt a pop and a brief burning pain in her left knee. On attempting to stand, the knee "gave out." She did not hit her head and has no neck pain. She had full memory of the event. She has an allergy to codeine, takes ibuprofen for headaches, has never injured the knee before, and has no significant past medical history. Her last meal was twenty minutes ago. The glissade was at the end of a ten-day backcountry trip with only a half-mile to go.

O: The instructor was found sitting upright in a stable position with the left knee flexed. She was fully alert, and warm and reasonably dry. She had no neck tenderness. The left knee was tender but not swollen, deformed, or discolored. She was able to flex and extend the knee fully with little discomfort. Distal CSM was intact. There was no other obvious injury. Vital signs at 13:20 were normal.

A: Unstable injury (possible fracture) left knee

A': Distal ischemia due to swelling

P: The knee was splinted with a snowshoe, and an improvised litter was fashioned from Ensolite pads and nylon webbing. Despite her embarrassment, the woman was carried the last half-mile to the road. Distal CSM was monitored by asking her if she could feel and wiggle her toes inside her boots.

Discussion: Although the temptation to limp the last half-mile was very strong, the patient agreed to the appropriate treatment. This injury fit the criteria for unstable injury because of the history of a pop during injury and the instability experienced afterward. This case is typical of a ligament rupture.

Case Study

S: A seventeen-year-old girl caught her right index finger between loose rocks during a descent of a scree slope fifteen miles from the trailhead. She was able to dislodge herself but complained of immediate pain. Shortly afterward she became dizzy and nauseated. The group leader climbed back up to examine the girl. Witnesses told him that she did not fall and was not struck by anything. She has no allergies, is not on medication, and has no significant past medical history. She had breakfast one hour ago. She had been walking without difficulty prior to the accident and was well rested and hydrated. The rock was stable, but the weather was cool and windy.

O: The patient was found lying against a large rock. She was disoriented, pale, and sweaty. The tip of the right index finger was swollen and very tender, with a superficial abrasion of the skin. There was no other injury. Her vital signs at 09:30 were: BP: unknown; P: 64; R: 24; S: pale, cool, moist; T: feels cool; C: V on AVPU with confusion and disorientation, improving.

A: 1. Fracture tip of right index finger

2. Skin wound, not high risk

3. Acute Stress Reaction

A': 1. Infection of abrasion right index finger.

P: The finger was immersed in clean cold water to irrigate the abrasion and relieve pain. The patient was encouraged to lie in a sleeping bag and calm down. Her vital signs rechecked at 10:00 were normal. The finger was splinted by taping it to the third finger with a gauze pad and antibiotic ointment between the fingers.

The girl was instructed to keep the finger elevated as much as possible and to use cool soaks for swelling and pain relief during rest stops. The wound was to be irrigated and the dressing changed daily. She was cautioned about the signs and symptoms of infection and instructed to check circulation and sensation at the fingertip frequently. She would be referred to medical care, if necessary, when the group reached the road in three days.

Discussion: Although this patient was displaying very frightening signs and symptoms immediately after the injury, there was no mechanism to explain it except ASR. The changes in level of consciousness and mental status rapidly resolved with rest, reassurance, and pain relief, leaving only an unhappy girl with a sore finger.

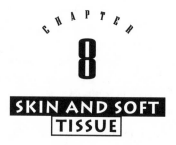

CHAPTER 8

SKIN AND SOFT TISSUE

Laceration of the skin is one of the most common reasons that students are evacuated from their solo experiences at the Hurricane Island Outward Bound School in Maine. The wounds are almost always caused by a slip of the knife blade while rendering some indispensable tool or work of art from a stubborn piece of driftwood. These injuries occur not for lack of preparation and precaution but rather because the creative spirit seems to get the better of the student's common sense.

To reduce the bloodletting, instructors have used every technique from giving detailed whittling lessons to no-whittling policies to outright banning of knives. But I like the creative spirit and believe the knife to be the most necessary of tools. I tend to favor instruction and precaution, and a good talk on wound care.

Students carry into the field with them everything they need to care for minor wounds. This consists of their own two hands, fresh water, soap, and clean gauze dressings. Their primary goal is to assist the body's own defensive and healing mechanisms. Definitive care, such as suturing (stitches), can be performed hours or days later if necessary.

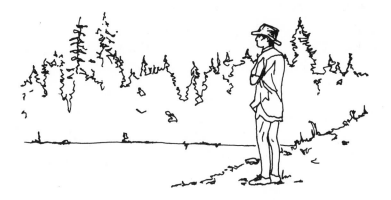

STRUCTURE AND FUNCTION

The skin is the largest of the body's organs. It performs the remarkable function of separating the flora and fauna of the outside environment from the sterile temperature- and chemical-sensitive internal organs. Most of the time it does a pretty good job, considering that it's less than a quarter of an inch thick.

Between the skin and underlying bone, joints, and organs is soft tissue, which includes fat, muscle, and connective tissue as well as the small vessels and nerves found in these layers. Problems begin when the protective outer layer of skin is damaged and the soft tissue beneath is exposed. This allows fungi, bacteria, and other microorganisms to invade the unprotected tissue and vital body fluids to escape.

SKIN AND SOFT-TISSUE PROBLEMS

WOUNDS

A wound is any injury that disrupts the skin. It can be superficial or deep. It can also involve structures other than soft tissue, such as bone, major nerves and vessels, and internal organs. Wounds come in a fascinating variety of types, but for field purposes we'll put them in four manageable groups:

LACERATION AND AVULSION.

The skin is divided (laceration) or sliced or torn away (avulsion). Either wound may be superficial or deep. There may be an "avulsion flap" still attached. The wound may also include some crushed and dead tissue.

AMPUTATION.

A complete segment of an extremity is lost, such as a finger or arm. Bleeding may be severe. The amputated part may sometimes be reattached several hours after injury.

SHALLOW WOUNDS.

Superficial burns and abrasions can disrupt the skin but do not penetrate through into the soft tissue.

PUNCTURE WOUNDS.

Skin disruption is minimal, but the injury extends into the soft tissue. The object that causes the puncture drags bacteria and other foreign material into the wound, almost invariably causing infection.

All wounds damage blood vessels and cause bleeding. The body can stop this blood loss by first automatically constricting blood vessels at the injury site to reduce blood flow. A clot then begins to form, and if it is left undisturbed it can bring bleeding to a halt within fifteen minutes. Serious bleeding problems can develop when injured vessels are numerous or very large. Severe blood loss (major circulatory system problem) can occur before the clotting mechanism seals the wound.

After the blood loss has been stopped, the slower process of wound repair begins. The initial stages of natural wound cleansing occur over a period of several days. The clot dries at the surface, forming a natural bandage in the form of a scab. Underlying tissue is further protected by the process of inflammation, which forms a protective barrier below.

Any contamination, such as dirt and bacteria, is moved to the surface as the wound drains. By the third or fourth day, the protective barriers are established and cleansing is well under way. The signs

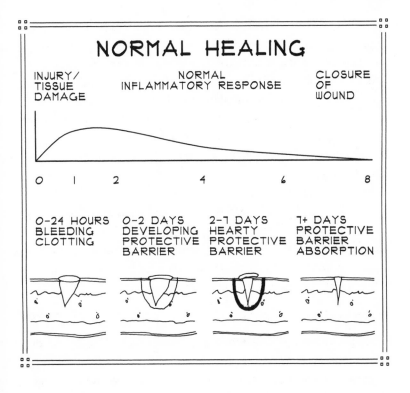

NORMAL HEALING

INJURY/ TISSUE DAMAGE	NORMAL INFLAMMATORY RESPONSE	CLOSURE OF WOUND

0   1   2   4   6   8

0-24 HOURS BLEEDING CLOTTING	0-2 DAYS DEVELOPING PROTECTIVE BARRIER	2-7 DAYS HEARTY PROTECTIVE BARRIER	7+ DAYS PROTECTIVE BARRIER ABSORPTION

of normal inflammation—redness, warmth, swelling, and pain—begin to subside as the protective barrier continues to grow stronger.

After six to eight days the wound is very resistant to new outside contamination. As inflammation subsides, wound edges migrate together and form a scar where they meet. Reinjury or excessive movement or wetting of the wound area during the early stages of healing can disrupt the barrier effect, allowing infection and delaying healing. This can be a real problem at sea, where staying dry and clean is especially difficult. You must be persistent and creative in protecting a wound in these conditions.

If the protective mechanisms are overwhelmed, invading bacteria can pass through the protective barrier into surrounding tissues. If the body's immune system is unable to control them, bacteria can reproduce rapidly, causing an infection. In an attempt to reestablish the barrier, the body increases local inflammation. Pus develops as the cellular debris and edema fluid accumulates. This combination of processes produce the early signs and symptoms of infection. If these symptoms affect only the immediate area of the wound, the infection is considered "local." If the infection spreads, it will ultimately enter the general circulation and be considered a "systemic" infection, sometimes called blood poisoning. The body responds with systemic inflammation that produces a generalized redness, fever, and pain. Patients with systemic infection can become very sick. Fortunately, this rarely happens as a complication of skin wounds in healthy people.

Some wounds are more prone to infection than others and are labeled "high risk." These wounds, which require more care and earlier medical attention, include puncture wounds and wounds involving joints and other complex structures as well as wounds that are dirty or involve crushed or dead tissue.

ASSESSMENT OF WOUNDS.

Although wounds, like fractures, are sometimes obvious and dramatic, they are rarely life-threatening in themselves. Start by looking for associated major body system problems and then move on to the wound itself, checking for evidence of high-risk factors.

High-Risk Wounds

Dirty wounds. Injuries with imbedded foreign material such as gravel, sawdust, or clothing fibers harbor bacteria that is difficult to dislodge.

Ragged wounds. Wounds in which there is crushed, shredded, or dead tissue, which provide growth medium for bacteria.

Complex wounds. Wounds that involve injuries to joints, tendons, and bones (open fractures) are difficult to clean adequately and are prone to serious infection.

Bite wounds. From humans or other animals. Mouths harbor a wide variety of virulent germs, and human bites are among the worst. Cat bites are pretty bad, too. Any wound exposed to human or animal saliva constitutes a bite wound.

Puncture wounds. A small opening in the skin with a wound track that extends through several layers deposits bacteria in areas that are unable to drain properly. These have a way of looking minor at first but becoming a big problem later. This is especially true when you drive a nail or thorn through a rubber sneaker or sandal into the bottom of your foot.

TREATMENT OF SOFT-TISSUE WOUNDS.

Treat the major body system problems *first!* Say your riding partner goes over the handlebars on a steep descent and you find him sitting on the trail with his face covered with blood from a small scalp laceration. Your first instinct is to wipe the blood away and help him up because you hate the sight of blood and want everything to look normal again. This is a perfectly natural reaction, but it's dead wrong. Do not forget that this is a mechanism for unstable cervical spine injury. Stabilize his neck until you are certain there is no spine injury or other major body system problem, *then* worry about the laceration.

Once your surveys are complete and any serious conditions are dealt with, you are ready to treat a soft-tissue wound. There are several steps to follow, and they apply to all wounds—big and small, clean and dirty, superficial and deep, and head to toe.

STOP EXTERNAL BLEEDING.

Direct pressure stops most bleeding, but to do it effectively you need to see where the blood is originating. Put on your latex gloves and glasses or goggles and cut away clothes, remove equipment, cut hair, or do whatever is necessary. If pressure is well aimed, most bleeding stops within fifteen minutes as the clotting mechanism is activated. If bleeding persists, it is usually because the pressure applied was too light or was poorly aimed. Remove the bandage, find the bleeding site, and try again. Once bleeding has stopped, the clot will keep it stopped unless disturbed.

Elevation helps reduce bleeding by reducing the blood pressure in the affected extremity.

Splinting helps reduce bleeding by preventing disruption of the clot by movement.

Ice, if available, will help constrict blood vessels in the area of the injury.

Tourniquets are used *only* if severe bleeding does not stop with direct pressure or there is no time to apply pressure effectively.

Pressure points are rarely useful in the field setting.

PREVENT INFECTION.

Long-term management (anything over two hours) requires early wound cleansing to help prevent infection. Cleansing a wound usually restarts some bleeding by disturbing the clot. If severe bleeding is a problem, leave the pressure dressing in place until bleeding is definitely stopped. *Do not attempt to clean wounds that are associated with life-threatening bleeding.*

Wash the skin around the wound with soap and water or disinfectant. Clean a wide area of skin, being careful not to allow soap or disinfectant into the wound itself.

Irrigate the wound with clean water (that is, water suitable for drinking). Rinse the wound by pouring water directly into the opening and allowing the water to run out by gravity. The greater the volume of water the better. You are flushing out debris and reducing the bacteria to levels that can be managed by the body's own defenses.

It is unnecessary and harmful to irrigate a wound with full-strength iodine preparations like Betadine or Povidone. Iodine kills both bacteria and body cells, leaving a partially sterilized wound lined with dead tissue. This can actually *increase* the chances of later infection. If water purification is required, use only a few drops of iodine in a quart of water, as you would to treat it for drinking.

Remove any imbedded debris from the wound. Anything that was not flushed out by irrigation should be removed manually. Brush the obvious junk out with a new toothbrush or other clean tool. A pair of tweezers is useful for removing pieces of gravel, or clothing that resists gentle persuasion. Cut off any torn pieces of tissue in the wound that are obviously ischemic, including pieces of skin and fat that are hanging or have turned blue or black.

Properly cleansing a wound can take quite a bit of time, especially if it's very dirty. Make sure the work area is well lit, you are comfortable, and you take the time to do a good job.

Cover the area with sterile dressings to prevent outside contamination of your nicely cleansed wound. Keep the dressings as clean and dry as possible. A sterile dressing can be covered with nonsterile bandages. Recleanse the wound and change dressings regularly, at least daily but even more frequently in wet or dirty conditions.

Leaving the wound open and allowing it to drain is important. Do not pull the wound edges together with tape (such as butterfly bandages) or try to suture it with dental floss. Closing a wound in the field is likely to create a nice demonstration of the obstruction and infection principle (see pages 7–8).

Splint the extremity if conditions and travel allow or if the wound is over a joint or an area subject to movement. This will minimize the breakdown of the protective barrier.

MEDICAL CARE.

High-risk wounds should receive early medical attention whenever possible, especially where open fracture is suspected. Infection generally takes a day or two to get going, so your ideal evacuation plan would have your patient out of the woods within forty-eight hours. During your walk out, pay careful attention to the wound, being especially vigilant about the removal of debris and irrigation. If your treatment is particularly effective, infection may never start.

Antibiotics given immediately offer some protection against the development of infection in high-risk wounds. If you are sailing or trekking days from medical care, carrying these drugs is a reasonable precaution. You should obtain a prescription and instructions from a medical practitioner.

Sutures (stitches) are used mainly to connect deep structures like tendons and ligaments and to close gaping wounds to reduce healing time and minimize scarring. Closing a wound with sutures requires training, experience, and a scrupulously clean environment. In the majority of cases it is not necessary or appropriate as a field treatment.

The kind of simple wound that might be successfully sutured by an inexperienced person doesn't need it anyway. Deep or complicated wounds need professional attention and should not be repaired by amateurs. Unless you really know what you are doing, leave the suture kit at home. Wound repair or scar revision can be safely delayed for days or weeks, if necessary.

Tetanus prophylaxis is an injectable vaccine given to anyone with an open wound who has not had a vaccination within ten years, or five years in the case of particularly dirty wounds. This is best done within twenty-four hours of injury. You can keep this from becoming a problem by getting a routine tetanus vaccination.

Monitor for signs of infection whether or not you choose to evacuate. You should also monitor the circulation, sensation, and movement (CSM) distal to the injury, as you would with a musculoskeletal problem. Bandages, splints, and swelling can create ischemia, so monitor carefully.

WOUND INFECTION

Infection is a possibility in any wound at any time during the healing process, but it is most likely to appear within two to four days after injury. It takes about that long for the typical skin-surface bacteria that have invaded the deeper layers to multiply and do enough damage to produce inflammation. But this time frame can vary widely depending on the health of the individual, the virulence of the bacteria, and the quality of wound care.

ASSESSMENT OF WOUND INFECTION.

In normal wound healing, pain, swelling, redness, and inflammation decrease quickly within the first two or three days. If the wound becomes infected, these signs and symptoms will begin to increase instead. Pus may be seen in the wound and may be accompanied by a foul odor.

When a wound does become infected, monitor it to see if it remains local or becomes systemic. The signs and symptoms of systemic infection include fever, nausea, generalized swelling of a larger area around the wound, and red streaks running toward the heart from the site of infection (inflammation of lymph ducts).

TREATMENT OF WOUND INFECTION.

Almost any wound that is becoming infected earns the status of high risk and should receive medical care. En route, you should continue regular cleaning and dressing changes. If the infected wound has been closed with tape or sutures, it should be opened and allowed to drain. Irrigate with water to remove pus. Do not squeeze

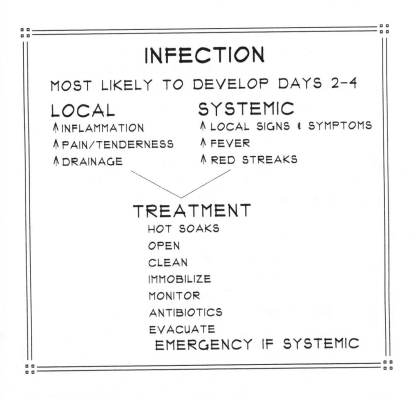

an infected wound or you will just drive bacteria through the protective barrier into healthy tissues.

Heat applications will increase circulation to the area to help the body fight the infection locally. Use only as much heat as you can comfortably stand against normal skin. Apply for thirty minutes at a time as often as five to six times a day.

Systemic infection is a medical emergency. Antibiotics should be started immediately, preferably by injection. Urgent evacuation is required. Septic shock (a form of vascular shock) is an anticipated problem.

IMPALED OBJECTS

An impaled object, like a knife or an ice axe, is best removed by a surgeon in a hospital. The ideal field treatment would stabilize the object in place while the patient is transported carefully to medical care. But in the backcountry this is nearly impossible. Trying to move the patient with the object in place will often risk more tissue damage than pulling it out. In most cases, an impaled object should be removed and the wound cleansed like any other.

Please note that impaled object removal doesn't work as in a classic Western. You don't just yank the arrow out while the patient bites on a bullet. Take your time and work the object slowly out of the tissue to minimize trauma. If it doesn't come easily, stop trying. Be prepared for bleeding. You may have to pack the wound with dressings afterwards to apply enough pressure in the right spot. On the other hand, it sometimes will be easier to control bleeding when the object is removed.

Remove Impaled Objects If:

1. The object cannot be stabilized or prevents safe transport.

2. The object is simple, safe, and easy to remove.

3. The object could obstruct the airway.

Abrasions (shallow wounds)

Abrasions are shallow wounds in which only the superficial layers of skin are scraped away. Because the deeper layers of the skin are still intact, healing can occur from the bottom up. This usually only takes a few days. Wound-care principles—stop bleeding and prevent infection—are the same.

Assessment of Abrasions.

Although there is usually some ground-in dirt and there may be thin flaps of skin hanging on at the wound margins, no fat or other soft tissue below the skin should be visible. The biggest problem with abrasions is the potential for infection. Also, you may notice that they always seem to happen in a place that's difficult to bandage.

Treatment of Abrasions.

As with lacerations, brush or pick out the foreign material and then irrigate the wound with clean water. Any hanging and dead skin should be trimmed away. Abrasions can be covered with antibiotic or antiseptic ointment and dressed with sterile gauze. Large abrasions or burns can be dressed with a clean cotton T-shirt, an article that you should carry in a plastic bag at the bottom of your backpack just for this purpose.

Long-term care is similar to that for lacerations. Clean and reapply a sterile dressing at least daily. You may use antibiotic ointment (such as Bacitracin or Neosporin) directly on the abrasion for pain relief and to help prevent infection. Generally, after about three to four days the abrasion will have healed enough to allow it to dry and scab over. If this is successful, keep it covered with dry dressings to prevent reinjury until it is well healed.

Burns

All burns are caused by heat transmitted from hot gases or objects or are produced by a chemical reaction between skin and a caustic substance. Burns can involve internal structures such as the respiratory system as well as skin itself.

ASSESSMENT OF BURNS.

For field management, we need to know the depth and extent of burns as well as their location. The extent is described in terms of body surface area (BSA), and critical locations include hands, feet, genitalia, and the respiratory system. Size estimates of irregular burns can be made using the patient's hand, which is about 1 percent of the body surface area, as a unit of measure.

The depth of burn refers to how deep the damage goes. It can be difficult to estimate the depth, particularly where different areas are burned to various degrees, but the following may serve as a rough guide:

Partial-Thickness Burns

First Degree. The skin integrity is not disrupted. Capillaries and nerves are intact. Inflammation occurs normally, with redness, pain, and warmth. This is the typical sunburn.

Second Degree. The skin surface is damaged, but the injury is limited to the outer layers. Capillaries are damaged, but deeper blood vessels and nerves are intact, allowing inflammation to produce blisters. There is fluid loss, redness, warmth, and pain.

Full-Thickness Burns

Third Degree. The full thickness of the skin is damaged. Capillaries, blood vessels, and nerves are destroyed. Normal inflammation cannot occur, and as a result blisters do not develop. The burned area may appear charred black, or gray. The area may not be painful due to loss of nerves. Small third-degree burns may appear to be less serious than they really are because of this.

As with other injury, look first for potentially life-threatening problems, usually in the form of volume shock and respiratory distress. High-risk burns are those that are likely to involve significant anticipated problems due to the potential for major body system involvement, pain, infection, or scar formation.

RESPIRATORY BURNS.

Burned respiratory passages will develop the same inflammation, blisters, and fluid loss that is seen on the skin. Respiratory burns should be suspected in any case where the patient was exposed to hot gases or steam, especially while trapped in a closed space. Signs and symptoms include singed facial hair, burned lips, sooty sputum, and persistent cough.

Respiratory distress is the anticipated problem and will develop as pulmonary fluid builds up in the lungs and swelling and obstruction occurs in the airways (see Chapter 5). Like any other swelling, it can develop quickly, or slowly over a period of days. This is a serious problem: Over 20 percent of respiratory burn patients die.

High-Risk Burns

1. Any respiratory involvement.

2. Second-degree burns of the face, genitalia, or hands.

3. Burns of any degree greater than 10 percent BSA. These burns have the potential to cause volume shock: The capillaries in burned skin can leak a tremendous amount of fluid.

4. Any third-degree burns.

5. Chemical burns. It can be difficult to fully arrest the burning process, because some chemicals react with the skin; damage can continue for hours afterward.

6. Electrical Burns. Skin damage may be minor, but electrical current can cause extensive injury to internal organs and tissues.

7. Burns associated with other serious injury.

8. Burns of very young or old patients.

TREATMENT OF BURNS.

It is imperative to stop the burning process. The first step in the management of burns is to immediately remove the heat. The fastest way to do this is to immerse the patient or injured part in water, which also serves to relieve pain. Be careful when dealing with larger burns, however, because you can make your patient hypothermic as a side effect of your good intentions. If the burn is greater than about 10 percent of the body surface area, limit your cooling to only a few minutes.

In chemical burns, continued irrigation with water will not only cool the area but will help remove the chemical itself. Irrigation should continue for at least thirty minutes.

EVACUATE HIGH-RISK BURNS.

If burns have the potential to cause life-threatening major body system problems, use Basic Life Support techniques and plan an emergency evacuation. With large burns, respiratory distress and shock are common. Any respiratory burn should be carefully monitored and evacuated without waiting for the development of severe symptoms.

CLEANSE THE BURN.

If the burn is not a life-threatening emergency, treat it like a minor abrasion, cleansing and dressing it with an antibiotic ointment. This can be done in conjunction with the application of cool soaks for pain relief. Continue to treat as you would any open wound. If the burn falls under the category of high risk, plan to have the patient to medical care within about forty-eight hours, if possible.

BLISTERS

MECHANISM OF INJURY.

Blisters, like the kind you get on your feet while hiking, are really burns caused by friction-generated heat. Your boots and socks rub against your skin, the damage results in leaky capillaries and swelling, and there you are: You not only have a skin injury to treat but a transportation problem as well. Keep walking on it and you will need a ride out of the woods just as surely as if you'd broken your leg.

ASSESSMENT OF BLISTERS.

Blisters progress through three stages. They begin with "hot spots," progress to blisters filled with sterile fluid, and then break to become contaminated superficial wounds. The stage at which you confront them and your logistical situation will determine your treatment. Generally, blisters act just like other shallow wounds.

TREATMENT OF BLISTERS.

Hot spots are where you begin to feel discomfort. You know something is wrong in your left boot, but you're only ten minutes into the hike and you don't want to stop yet. I don't blame you, especially if the black flies are bad. But stop you must. Outward Bound instructors, at least the smart ones, routinely stop their groups early in their first hike to do a foot check and give a talk on blister prevention.

Stop the friction immediately and you can prevent a blister from forming. Change your socks, fiddle with your laces, or cover the sore area with smooth surface tape, gel dressings, or moleskin. You can also apply antibiotic ointment to lubricate the area and reduce friction. Whatever time it takes to cool the hot spot will be well worth it in the long run. If blisters do develop, the important fact to remember early on is that a blister is a sterile wound until it breaks. Whenever we can, we like to keep it unbroken. Like in an abrasion, in an intact blister the lower layers of the skin are still unbroken, so the wound will heal quickly from below. Small blisters can be covered with gel dressing. Larger ones will usually cause some degree of disability unless you can take the original pressure off.

If the blister has formed in a bad spot, such as the back of your heel, you may have to drain it in order to be able to walk. Although you will be converting a closed and sterile wound into an open one, you can minimize the risk of infection by following a few simple procedures. First, as with other wounds, cleanse the skin around and over the blister with soap and water. Sterilize a needle or sharp knife blade over a flame or with alcohol. Make a tiny hole in the blister at its lower margin and allow the fluid to drain out. Leave the skin over the blister intact to act as its own sterile dressing. Cover the area with antibiotic ointment and dress it as you might a hot spot. As with any open wound, it must be cleansed and dressed daily and monitored for signs of infection.

Open blisters occur when a blister has broken and become non-sterile. An open blister should be treated like an abrasion. Cut away the dead skin and irrigate to remove debris, then cover the wound with antibiotic ointment and sterile dressings. Cleanse daily and monitor for infection. Fix the source of friction with padding or tape.

Case Study—Wounds

S: A twenty-three-year-old student on a research vessel was struck on the head by a swinging davit when a winch cable snapped while hauling a plankton net. He was found sitting on deck with a large and freely bleeding laceration across the top of his head.

He remembered everything about the event. He denied neck pain and had no other complaints. He denied allergies, was taking no medications, was well fed and warm, had no significant medical history, and was up to date on his tetanus vaccination.

The vessel was in the Gulf Stream approximately three hundred miles southeast of Cape Cod. The weather was mild but expected to deteriorate over the following twenty-four hours.

O: Awake, oriented, cooperative man holding a blood-soaked kerchief on his head. Blood covered his left shoulder and chest, and there was a large pool on the deck. He has no neck deformity or tenderness, has full range of motion and normal sensation of extremities with no numbness or tingling. The scalp had a 4-centimeter laceration, clean and straight, through the skin and subcutaneous tissue to the skull. No depression or bone fragments could be seen or felt. Vital signs at 18:05 were: BP: 112/78; P: 88; R: 16; C: awake and oriented; T: normal; S: normal color and temperature.

A: 1. Scalp wound

A': Wound infection (unlikely)

P: 1. Direct pressure to stop bleeding. Clean surrounding scalp and hair with soap and water. Irrigate wound with water. Dress with sterile dressings and a hat to hold them in place. Monitor and redress twice a day. Follow-up with physician in Bermuda during planned port call in three days.

Discussion: The scalp did just what it was designed to do. By slipping and tearing, it absorbed enough of the force of the impact to protect the skull and brain. There was no head injury, just a scalp wound. As is common with the scalp, bleeding was profuse but easily controlled with direct pressure. Although there looked like a lot of blood, vital signs showed that not enough was lost to produce shock. Because of the rich blood supply to the scalp, even deep scalp wounds usually heal well with a very low incidence of infection. There was no emergency here.

Unfortunately, bloody scalp wounds generate a lot of unnecessary anxiety and precipitate a lot of dangerous evacuations. Coast Guard and navy records are full of long flights in bad weather to rescue patients just like this one. Whatever benefit this might have must be weighed against sometimes substantial risks. If you think that your life is exciting, talk to a helicopter pilot about in-flight refueling at night.

SECTION IV

Toxins

and

Allergies

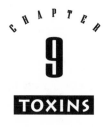

9

TOXINS

Toxic substances can produce systemic effects, local effects, or both, and affect more than one body system. The cause and effect relationship may be fairly obvious or quite confusing. Fortunately, the generic treatments can be applied successfully even when the exact toxin is not known. The major concern is how the body is reacting to the toxic exposure and what you can do to lessen symptoms and prevent serious injury.

Studying detailed descriptions of various poisonous plants, insects, spiders, snakes, and other creatures is interesting but not often helpful. Specific identification is difficult, even with a color key and a lot of experience. Although you should try to obtain as much information from the scene as possible, the investigation should not delay treatment or endanger rescuers.

GENERAL PRINCIPLES FOR ALL TOXINS

SYSTEMIC VS. LOCAL EFFECTS

Systemic toxins are those that affect the body as a whole. They may be ingested, injected, inhaled, or absorbed through the skin. Some common examples include mushrooms, bee stings, carbon monoxide, and poison ivy.

Local toxins affect only the immediate area of contact. Some toxins have both systemic and local effects. Examples are poisonous snakebites and inhaled gases that burn the respiratory system and are absorbed into the general circulation.

GENERAL ASSESSMENT OF TOXIC EXPOSURE.

Don't get distracted by trying to identify the toxin. Worry first about the effect it is having on the body. Look for signs of respiratory distress, shock, or changes in brain function. Check for swelling and ischemia. Toxins can cause problems with all three of the major body systems. Like the generic treatment for respiratory distress, there are generic principles for the treatment of toxic exposure.

GENERAL PRINCIPLES OF TREATMENT IN TOXIC EXPOSURE

REMOVE AND DILUTE

INGESTED TOXINS.

Induce vomiting, but only in patients who are conscious and alert and able to protect their own airways. This treatment should be restricted to poisonings where the toxin is known, such as a drug overdose or poisonous plant ingestion. Do not induce vomiting when the ingested substance is corrosive or a petroleum product.

Induction of vomiting is best done within the first hour after ingestion but may be effective several hours after ingestion. Give one to two tablespoons (15–30 cubic centimeters) syrup of ipecac orally, followed by two cups of water. The patient will vomit within twenty minutes. Be sure that the patient is positioned to prevent airway obstruction. After all vomiting has stopped, give activated charcoal (25–50 grams) mixed with water. This will absorb and hold the remaining toxin for excretion.

In the backcountry setting, induced vomiting can create its own problems, which may be worse than the toxic exposure. Persistent vomiting can make the patient become dehydrated, fatigued, and make any evacuation much more difficult. If you are worried that vomiting may confer more risk than benefit, give only the water and activated charcoal.

INHALED TOXINS.

Move the patient to clean air. Provide the generic treatment for respiratory distress (see page 48).

SKIN AND SOFT-TISSUE TOXINS.

Cleanse the area as you would a skin wound. Irrigate copiously with water.

ANTIDOTE

Effective antidotes are not always available and their use is limited to cases where the toxin is known, such as in snakebite or certain drugs. If possible, contact a poison control center for specific treatments.

BASIC LIFE SUPPORT

With time, most toxins are excreted or metabolized by the body so treatment is aimed at supporting body systems and treating problems as they develop until the toxin is removed or can be neutralized by an antidote. This generic approach is also effective when toxins are mixed or unknown.

SPECIFIC TOXINS—MARINE TOXINS, SNAKEBITE, INSECTS, AND ARACHNIDS

MARINE TOXINS

There are three ways to get poisoned in the marine environment: by spines, nematocysts, and fangs.

Spines are used for defense by a number of marine organisms, and some are coated with toxins or are able to inject toxins. Examples include stingrays, scorpion fish, catfish, and some sea urchins. The species found in waters around North America generally produce only localized pain and swelling. In Pacific waters, particularly around Australia, the organisms are a lot more dangerous.

The sting of a poisonous ray, urchin, or fish is easy to distinguish from a nontoxic puncture. The pain caused by the wound itself is minimal compared to the discomfort caused by the toxin, which increases quickly with time. The barbed stinger or spine will often remain in the wound.

Nematocysts are structures in the stinging parts of jellyfish, corals, and anemones that fire something resembling a microscopic harpoon when touched. These harpoons then inject a chemical toxin into the skin. The sensation is like a thousand tiny bee stings, a feeling that is typical with the sting from coral, jellyfish, and anemones.

The pain, surprise, and indignation one feels is usually followed by a rapid increase in the level of discomfort. As you wipe at the source of the pain, you stimulate the firing of more nematocysts and cause yourself more pain. Often jellyfish are broken up by surf, and the nematocyst-bearing tentacles are floating free and almost invisible in the water. Swimming into one can be a very frightening experience because the stinging sensation continues, and you can't see what's causing it.

Fangs in ocean-going creatures are poisonous only in a few species of sea snake. They are quite deadly, with a toxin that causes systemic as well as local effects. It is well worth seeking local advice about these creatures in areas where they are found.

TREATMENT OF MARINE TOXINS

SPINE INJURY.

The toxin is deactivated by heat. Immerse the affected part in water as hot as is tolerable for thirty to ninety minutes, or until the pain is relieved. Treat the wound itself as any puncture wound. By removing the spine or stinger, if possible, you will decrease the chances of infection.

NEMATOCYST INJURY.

Wash off the nematocysts with salt water, then scrape the skin in one direction, downward, with a firm-edged object like the back of your knife blade. Do *not* rinse in fresh water to remove nematocysts, because this will stimulate them to fire. Soak or bathe the affected part in alcohol or vinegar for thirty minutes, or until the pain is relieved. This will deactivate the remaining nematocysts. Powder and shave the skin to remove remaining nematocysts if pain persists.

SYSTEMIC EFFECTS.

Systemic effects are usually minimal but must be anticipated. These can involve all major body systems, but respiratory distress is the most prominent symptom. Fortunately, it requires a massive exposure to most marine toxins to have significant systemic effects. Basic Life Support, wound care, and evacuation for antivenin treatment may be wise in certain specific cases involving toxic fish and mollusks, especially in South Pacific waters. Consult local authorities about the area in which you plan to travel.

SNAKEBITE

In North America there are only two types of poisonous snakes to worry about, unless you happen to work in a zoo: pit vipers and coral snakes. The pit vipers, which include rattlesnakes, copperheads, and cottonmouths, have essentially the same toxin. It is mostly a hemotoxin, which causes primarily local swelling and tissue damage. The degree of systemic involvement depends on the dose injected and the general health of the patient. Some pit vipers, notably the Mojave rattlesnake, have a larger component of systemic neurotoxin than others, which can cause some nervous system symptoms.

Coral snake venom is primarily systemic and affects the nervous system. It can take several hours for symptoms to arise. It requires some work on a person's part to be bitten by a coral snake, a small-mouthed, shy creature. Victims are usually children.

ASSESSMENT OF SNAKEBITE.

Identification of the snake may be helpful but is not required for treatment. Pit vipers leave one or two fang marks. If venom has been injected (envenomation) there will be immediate swelling and pain. If no venom was injected, the pain will be only what you'd expect from the small puncture wounds and won't immediately get worse. It is useful to note that in about 40 percent of poisonous snakebites, venom is never injected. Of course, Acute Stress Reaction may make the distinction difficult to discern right after being bitten.

Because of its small fangs, the coral snake will have to chew its way into your skin to successfully inject venom. The effects may be delayed for several hours. Because of this delay, the bite of a suspected coral snake must always be considered envenomated. Symptoms of coral snake bite include tingling of the extremity possibly progressing to the whole body. The patient may develop respiratory distress if the nervous system is affected.

TREATMENT OF SNAKEBITE. BASIC LIFE SUPPORT.

Antivenin is usually restricted to a hospital, because it can cause life-threatening allergic reactions in rare cases. It is most effective when given during the first four hours after a bite but can be given up to several days following the bite and still have some benefit. Pit viper antivenin is effective for all of the members of that family of snakes, be it a rattler, copperhead, or cottonmouth. The presence of fang marks is enough to identify the bite of a pit viper. Coral snake antivenin, however, is specific to that species.

Antibiotics are usually given to prevent infection. As a puncture and bite wound, snakebite certainly qualifies as high risk, with or without envenomation.

Transport the patient as quickly as possible to antivenin. Immediately following the bite of a snake thought to be poisonous, evacuation should be started without delay. Walking your patient out may be the fastest way to go, and this is fine unless severe symptoms prevent it. Your evacuation can always be slowed down or canceled if it becomes obvious that envenomation did not occur or the snake was not poisonous.

Splint the affected extremity if possible.

Expect swelling. Remove constricting items such as rings, bracelets, and clothing from the bitten extremity to prevent ischemia.

Do not apply tourniquets, pressure dressing, ice packs, or use "cut and suck" snakebite kits. These are ineffective and dangerous. Some authorities recommend the use of a constricting band to reduce the lymphatic drainage in the bitten extremity without compromising blood flow, but these bands are difficult to control and may result in more damage.

INSECTS AND ARACHNIDS

Insect and arachnid (spiders, scorpions) toxins are encountered in a couple of different ways. Venom may be injected by a stinger or specialized mouth part as the animal—wasp, fire ant, spider, or scorpion—attempts to defend itself or warn you away from a nest. The sting is meant to hurt, and it usually does.

More commonly, the skin becomes irritated in reaction to substances used by a feeding insect. One such toxin prevents clotting of blood, and many insects inject a local anesthetic to reduce the pain caused by the bite, at least for as long as they're feeding. Examples include black flies, moose flies, mosquitoes, gnats, and most of the rest of the insect population of North America (or so it seems).

ASSESSMENT AND TREATMENT OF INSECT AND ARACHNID TOXINS.

Local reaction to these toxins can be severe but involve only the extremity or immediate area of the bite or sting. There may be some degree of Acute Stress Reaction, which must be distinguished from systemic effects. Local reactions are treated for comfort with cool soaks, elevation, and rest. Aspirin, ibuprofen, or other anti-inflammatory pain medications will help, as will diphenhydramine or other antihistamines.

SYSTEMIC REACTION.

Anaphylaxis is an allergic reaction to venom or other substances whereby the whole body is affected by rapid generalized swelling, hives, respiratory distress, nausea, and shock. This is a true medical emergency, often requiring epinephrine and antihistamines to save the patient's life. The indications for and use of these drugs are discussed in Chapter 10.

Toxin load is the term applied to the cumulative effects of multiple stings or bites. Toxin loading, which can produce systemic effects that may be delayed up to twenty-four hours, is common in black fly country in the spring and early summer. Symptoms include fever, fatigue, headache, and nausea. This is not an allergic reaction: The generalized swelling, respiratory distress, and other signs of anaphylaxis are absent.

Toxin load is usually no emergency. Observe for twenty-four hours. Give aspirin, ibuprofen, or other anti-inflammatory pain reliever for comfort. Watch for signs of infection at the site of insect bites. Keep the patient well hydrated and protected from excessive cooling or heating.

Case Study—Toxins

S: A sixteen-year-old male on a canoe expedition in the Florida Everglades was bitten on the right arm by a four-foot snake as he was trying to throw it off his lap. It apparently dropped off an overhead branch. In the ensuing confusion, the snake escaped overboard. The boy was unable to describe it other than as dark in color and very fast. He complained of pain in the mid-right forearm. The boy had no allergies and was not taking any medication. He had no past history of significant medical problems and had eaten breakfast three hours previously. There was no other recent trauma or illness.

It was midmorning, the sky was clear, and the temperature was about 75 degrees. The expedition was approximately seven miles from the ranger station at Flamingo.

O: The patient was awake but pale and anxious. He had two small puncture wounds on his right forearm. There was no swelling or discoloration. The area was tender to the touch. Distal CSM was intact. There were no other injuries. Vital signs at 10:15 were: BP: unavailable; P: 120; R: 24; T: appears normal; S: pale; C: Awake and anxious.

A: 1. Snakebite, possibly venomous

    2. Acute Stress Reaction

A': 1. Swelling and ischemia in the right arm

    2. Allergic or other systemic effects of injected toxin

P: The right arm was put at rest with a sling made from the boy's T-shirt and a diaper pin. The boy was placed amidships in a canoe paddled by two other people, and evacuation to the ranger station began immediately. Vital sign and CSM checks were done every fifteen minutes. A brief SOAP note was written and sent with the patient.

Discussion: At the time of the first set of vital signs, the boy was found to be awake, oriented, and relatively calm. Vital signs were near normal. He complained only of slight pain in the arm. A power boat was flagged down to complete the evacuation. On arrival at the ranger station forty minutes later, the boy's condition appeared normal. It was determined that no envenomation had occurred, even though the bite was probably from a water moccasin. He was treated for puncture wounds at a local clinic and returned to the expedition the next day. The evacuation of this patient was appropriate, even though it turned out that there was no emergency. Had the snake actually injected venom, the patient would have been moving in the direction of antivenin and Advanced Life Support, had it been necessary.

10

ANAPHYLAXIS

Anaphylaxis is a severe systemic allergic reaction to a foreign material that enters the circulating blood. It can be caused by substances in food that are absorbed in the intestine, substances inhaled and absorbed through the lungs, or substances injected into the skin, such as bee venom. The reaction to substances eaten with food may be delayed due to the time it takes to digest them, but anaphylaxis is usually immediate (within a few seconds or minutes) when it involves inhaled or injected material.

ASSESSMENT OF ANAPHYLAXIS

The signs and symptoms of anaphylaxis are caused by widespread blood vessel dilation and tissue swelling of all body surfaces. This can produce life-threatening vascular shock and swelling and obstruction of the airway, and death can occur in a matter of minutes in severe reactions. Most patients have a history of allergy to the substance involved, but this is not always the case. The severity of past reactions is not a reliable indicator of what will happen in the present.

In true anaphylaxis the patient may complain of hot, burning, itchy skin and suffer from nausea, vomiting, and even diarrhea.

There will be some degree of respiratory distress. The patient may feel weakness and disorientation with the onset of shock. Vital signs are consistent with shock due to widespread blood vessel dilation and respiratory distress due to lower-airway constriction (see Chapters 4 and 5).

Vital Signs in Anaphylaxis

P: Increased

R: Increased with distress, wheezing if severe

BP: Decreased if severe

C: Anxious, confused; V,P, or U if severe

S: Flushed, with hives, general swelling

T: Unchanged

The Focused History and Physical Exam will reveal generalized swelling of the face, eyes, tongue, and skin. The appearance of hives is a key indicator. Do not confuse anaphylaxis with a severe *local* reaction, such as a swollen arm after a bee sting. The anaphylaxis patient will almost always have altered mental status, and may not be responsive. It is also easy to mistake anaphylaxis for seizure or Acute Stress Reaction, so be especially careful in your assessment, because it can be difficult if there is no history to go on.

TREATMENT OF ANAPHYLAXIS

Provide Basic Life Support as you would for any patient with shock and respiratory distress. However, specific treatment with drugs is required to reverse severe reactions, and it should be administered immediately, before the reaction has progressed to a critical condition.

The drug most frequently used is injectable epinephrine, which is the synthetic version of the hormone adrenaline. Epinephrine reverses the symptoms of severe reactions by causing systemic constriction of blood vessels. The drug is supplied specifically for this purpose in the form of bee-sting kits that contain a preloaded hypodermic syringe. The easiest to use is the Epipen, which automatically injects the right dose when pressed firmly against the skin. These devices are available only by prescription. Any member of your group who has a known insect allergy should obtain one of these kits and instructions for its use before going into the backcountry.

Be aware that epinephrine does not remove or neutralize the foreign material that caused the reaction. It is possible to see a rebound reaction with the reappearance of symptoms minutes or hours later, when the epinephrine wears off. Multiple doses may be necessary.

Antihistamines are also used in the treatment of anaphylaxis. These drugs do not immediately reverse blood vessel dilation or vascular shock like epinephrine but can help prevent further reaction to the histamine and prevent rebound effect. Any antihistamine is helpful, even the stuff in your over-the-counter cold medication, of which Benadryl (diphenhydramine) is the most common. In the emergency room, Benadryl is often given immediately after an epinephrine injection. That way, the Benadryl can take over just about the time the epinephrine is wearing off.

Because the effects of epinephrine are temporary, evacuation should be instituted at once. If the patient has recovered from the event, it need not be an emergency. Careful monitoring for rebound reaction is crucial. Also, be aware that a second exposure to the same foreign material can cause an even more severe reaction.

SECTION V

Environmental

Medicine

11

PROBLEMS WITH
BODY CORE TEMPERATURE

The core of the human body operates most efficiently at or very near a temperature of 98.6 degrees Fahrenheit (37.2 Centigrade). Even a small change in either direction can adversely affect the normal chemical reactions that are part of all body processes. Fortunately, a healthy body and intelligent mind can control its internal temperature by balancing heat loss and heat production against the challenges of environmental conditions. You put on or shed clothing, seek the shade when you're hot or lie in the sun like a lizard when you're cold. You curl up to preserve heat or spread yourself out to get rid of it. Your intelligence and freedom of movement are important factors in striking the balance.

Much of the process is, however, unconscious. The body's compensatory mechanisms constrict blood vessels in the skin to keep heat in the core or dilate them to radiate excess heat. Sweat glands release fluid to enhance cooling by evaporation. Shivering produces heat with involuntary exercise. Even though we can watch them work, these mechanisms are not under our direct control.

Problems with temperature regulation develop when the compensatory mechanisms fail due to injury, illness, accident, or ignorance. As you might have guessed, one of the first signs of abnormal core temperature is a change in consciousness and mental status. You rapidly lose your judgment and common sense, and from there the problems only get worse.

Hyperthermia and hypothermia are systemic problems involving too much heat or too little heat, respectively, in the body core. With each we can define three distinct stages. The first stage is the body's normal and healthy response to the environmental challenge. The second marks the failure of the compensatory mechanisms with mild changes in core temperature. The third stage represents a severe, life-threatening condition with complete loss of temperature regulation.

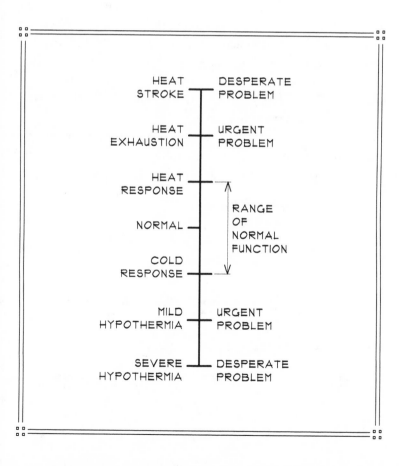

HYPERTHERMIA

HEAT CHALLENGE VS. PASSIVE HEAT LOSS AND ACTIVE HEAT LOSS

Both internal and external factors come into play when dealing with the challenges produced by heat. Inside your body, heat is constantly being produced as a by-product of metabolism and increases dramatically with exercise. Because your vital organs work best at a temperature of around 98.6 degrees Fahrenheit, the body will conserve only as much heat as it needs to keep it at that temperature and will get rid of the rest.

Your primary tool for dumping excess heat is the dilation of shell blood vessels and the production of sweat. As your body temperature rises, more blood is shunted to the skin where excess heat can radiate into the environment (passive heat loss). The process is dramatically enhanced by sweating, because water absorbs a tremendous amount of heat from the skin as it evaporates (active heat loss). This is a very efficient cooling system, as long as there is enough blood and sweat to keep it going.

The external factors in the heat challenge include not only the temperature of the surrounding environment but also the humidity of the air and exposure to wind. This directly affects the efficiency

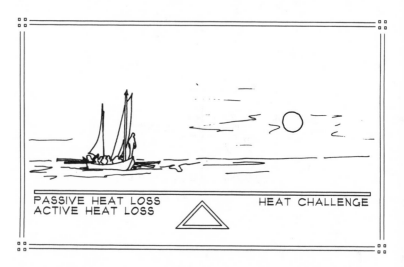

PASSIVE HEAT LOSS
ACTIVE HEAT LOSS
HEAT CHALLENGE

of the heat-loss mechanism. Moving air speeds evaporation and the conduction of heat away from the body, and dry air allows faster evaporation than humid air.

HEAT RESPONSE

It is a warm day and a group of friends are hiking. You are all sweating. Here we see the body's heat loss mechanism at work. The skin is vasodilated and fluid is being sacrificed at a prodigious rate. As long as the mechanisms for shedding heat can keep up with the heat challenge, the body temperature will remain normal. But pushing yourself or others out of balance is asking for trouble. Instead of overdoing it, follow common sense by reducing exercise, removing clothing, seeking shade, and replacing fluids. Also, be aware of your environment. Sweat can evaporate so quickly in dry climates that profuse sweating may go unnoticed until fluid loss is severe. In humid environments the amount of fluid lost to sweat will be much more obvious, because it runs into your eyes and drips off your nose because it can't evaporate.

When the signs of heat response are present, pay special attention to fluid replacement. It is important to realize that being thirsty is a relatively late sign of fluid depletion. By the time you feel thirst, your tank is already getting low. Drink *before* you become thirsty! A better sign of fluid status is urine output. You'll know that you're getting enough water if you are producing light yellow urine at your normal and healthy rate. If your urine is darker (more concentrated) and less frequent than you're used to, you will know that your body is trying to conserve water.

HEAT EXHAUSTION

This is the beginning of trouble. Heat exhaustion is actually early volume shock caused by dehydration. The term is a little misleading, however, because core temperature is not yet significantly elevated.

ASSESSMENT OF HEAT EXHAUSTION.

You will recognize the vital-sign pattern as mild compensated volume shock including the shell/core effect. In the backcountry, heat exhaustion is a serious problem that requires immediate treatment.

Vital Signs in Heat Exhaustion

BP: Normal or decreased

P: Increased

R: Increased

S: Variable; may be flushed or clammy

T: Normal or slightly elevated

C: Awake with mildly altered mental status

Urine output is decreased as the body seeks to conserve fluid.

General condition will be weak, thirsty, and nauseated. Vomiting is common.

TREATMENT OF HEAT EXHAUSTION.

Reduce the heat challenge by moving the patient into the shade. Stop physical exertion, fan the patient with fresh air, and assist evaporative cooling with water. The object is to stop the progression of volume shock by preventing further dehydration through sweating. Radical cooling, such as immersion in ice water, is not necessary.

Fluid replacement should begin immediately. Oral intake is usually adequate, but intravenous fluid is faster if available. Even if the patient is vomiting oral replacement is still possible by frequently giving fluid in small amounts. Look for normal urine production and normal mental status as an indication of adequate fluid volume. Without intravenous fluids it may take more than twelve hours to bring the dehydrated patient back to normal.

Replacing salt is a good idea following heavy sweating but is not necessary for emergency treatment. Salt, if you're worried about it, is provided by most foods. You can also make a reasonable rehydration drink by adding a pinch of salt and a pinch of sugar to a quart of water. Do not give salt tablets, which cause stomach irritation and vomiting.

HEAT STROKE

This is a life-threatening emergency requiring immediate field treatment. The body's heat loss mechanisms are overwhelmed by the heat challenge and the core temperature rises out of control to critical levels (greater than 105 degrees Fahrenheit). There is no time for delay. Once hyperthermia has reached this point, the chances of survival are not good.

ASSESSMENT OF HEAT STROKE.

There are unmistakable changes in level of consciousness. Severe mental status changes will rapidly lead to a drop on the AVPU scale. The skin may have the classic hot, red, and dry appearance, but this is not always the case. In the presence of an extreme heat challenge, a critical rise in core temperature can occur before the patient has time to become dehydrated, so the skin may be wet with sweat or clammy due to shock. This extreme heat challenge can be caused by anything from hiking all day in a hot environment to staying in a sauna for an extended period.

Regardless of the fluid status or how quick the onset, these heat stroke patients look very sick. The key indicators are a positive mechanism for hyperthermia, a high core temperature, and any changes in level of consciousness.

Vital Signs in Heat Stroke

BP: Variable to decreased

P: Increased

R: Increased

S: Variable; may be flushed or clammy or dry or sweaty

T: Severely elevated, above 105 degrees Fahrenheit

C: Changes in consciousness preceded by mental status changes (for instance, hallucinating or agitated). May have seizures.

TREATMENT OF HEAT STROKE.

Radical cooling is required. The best method we've heard about was developed by the Israeli army. Soldiers are stripped, suspended in a hammock, sprayed with a mist of water, and fanned with air. This technique makes maximum use of evaporative cooling.

If you're not equipped as well as the Israeli army, you can still pour whatever water you have onto the patient's skin and fan it vigorously. This method may be preferable to just dunking the patient in cold water, which will cause immediate vasoconstriction of the skin as well as prevent any cooling from evaporation. Dunking can also result in a rapid swing toward hypothermia if you're not careful. Look for an improvement in consciousness and mental status to determine the return to a more normal temperature.

Oral fluid replacement, besides being too slow, is impossible in the unresponsive patient. Intravenous replacement is clearly the treatment of choice, but the necessary equipment is not in everybody's backpack. Intravenous fluids are a top priority when and if Advanced Life Support services become available.

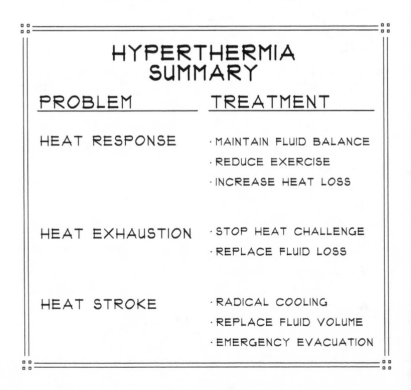

HYPERTHERMIA SUMMARY

PROBLEM	TREATMENT
HEAT RESPONSE	· MAINTAIN FLUID BALANCE · REDUCE EXERCISE · INCREASE HEAT LOSS
HEAT EXHAUSTION	· STOP HEAT CHALLENGE · REPLACE FLUID LOSS
HEAT STROKE	· RADICAL COOLING · REPLACE FLUID VOLUME · EMERGENCY EVACUATION

Basic Life Support is instituted as needed to preserve vital functions during cooling. The recovery of a heat stroke patient is dependent on quick, radical field treatment.

Evacuation is necessary even if you succeed in reducing the core temperature in time to save the patient. Heat stroke patients have suffered a severe injury and require treatment and observation in the hospital. Brain injury or shock are common. Emergency evacuation is certainly justified.

HYPOTHERMIA

COLD CHALLENGE VS. HEAT RETENTION AND HEAT PRODUCTION

Our good friend and colleague, John Haskins, is a superb Outward Bound instructor. John has spent plenty of time in small open boats off the coast of Maine, which has given him a lot of firsthand experience with hypothermia. No one could design a better laboratory than Maine for studying the effects of long-term exposure to cold and wet environments. As with hyperthermia, one of the first things to be affected by hypothermia is judgment and common sense. The fact that John keeps going back out there seems to prove this point.

The Maine coast is particularly good at providing all the elements of the cold challenge: a low ambient temperature; wetness in the form of rain, fog, and general high humidity; and wind. To counter the challenge, John uses passive heat retention in the form of insulation (fat and winter clothing) and constriction of the blood vessels in the skin to keep warmth in the body core (shell/core effect). He also reduces the area of his body exposed to heat loss by curling up in the bottom of the boat. By this time John is usually cold, shivering, and miserable.

He is quick to recognize the shell/core effect and his body's attempt to produce heat—he leaps to an oar and rows briskly to help with active heat production. His students think he's crazy, but this helps John feel better. He also knows that in order to produce heat, he needs calories to burn. This is a perfect excuse to eat something, which makes John feel much better. He may still be at sea and lost in the fog, but at least he's warm.

C O L D   R E S P O N S E

Here are the body's heat retention and heat production mechanisms at work. The shell/core effect reduces blood flow to the skin, reducing heat loss to the environment. There may be slight or obvious shivering as the body attempts to produce heat from muscular exercise. Because the compensation mechanisms are working, the core temperature is normal. The level of consciousness and mental status are normal. The skin will be pale and cool, with the person (not yet a patient) feeling uncomfortably cold.

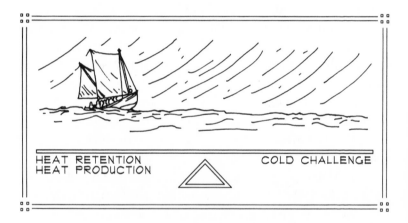

HEAT RETENTION
HEAT PRODUCTION
COLD CHALLENGE

Because the body is already using compensatory mechanisms to maintain core temperature, further changes in the environment or a limited food and fluid supply can overwhelm the body's ability to compensate, resulting in hypothermia. *Now* is the time to tip the balance back toward body warmth by reducing the cold challenge and increasing heat retention and production.

Beware of trying to produce heat without calories to burn. Living outside in a cold environment can require more than six thousand calories a day, so you obviously don't want to be on a diet or lying passively in cold bilge water. *Get into dry clothing, eat, and exercise!*

Another interesting phenomenon associated with the cold response is cold diuresis. This is the tendency of the body to produce more urine when shell/core compensation occurs. As blood is shunted into the core, the kidneys sense an increase in fluid volume in the central circulation and proceed to get rid of some of it.

Cold diuresis, and the logistics involved in obtaining fresh water in an extreme environment, can lead to fluid volume depletion. Normal volume is necessary for adequate heat production. Make the additional effort to keep yourself well hydrated.

Mild Hypothermia

The onset of hypothermia is more insidious than dramatic. Any idiot can diagnose hypothermia in someone who's been overboard in the gulf of Maine for forty minutes. Usually, however, hypothermia creeps up on you because you allow yourself or someone else to be just a little cold for a long time.

As cooling continues, passive heat retention and active heat production are overwhelmed by the cold challenge, and the body core temperature falls below 96 degrees Fahrenheit. This can occur rapidly, as in cold-water immersion, or slowly over hours or days. Hypothermia can often coexist with other problems or be a complication of trauma, intoxication, altitude sickness, or any other condition that reduces a person's resistance to the cold challenge.

Hypothermia can contribute to injury or death from other mechanisms. Most drowning, for example, occurs because the extremities become uncoordinated as the body shell cools when exposed to cold water. Hypothermia can lead to errors in judgment, resulting in a fall while rock climbing or going overboard while working on a slippery deck offshore. It must always be suspected when there is any problem in a cool setting.

Assessment of Mild Hypothermia.

In rapid onset cases (such as going overboard in cold water), the body's fuel stores of available calories have not been used up so there is often a radical difference in temperature between the cold body shell and the still relatively warm body core. In slow-onset cases, fuel stores are often depleted and the temperature difference between shell and core is not as dramatic. Such a gradual appearance of symptoms often makes recognition difficult.

The most obvious outward signs of mild hypothermia are mental status changes and shivering. The patient may be lethargic, withdrawn, confused, or exhibit personality changes. A normally pleasant crew member may become irritable and hostile. A person who is normally loud and unpleasant may become quiet and complacent (which is particularly dangerous because there will be tremendous temptation to leave him that way).

The skin of the hypothermic patient will be pale and cool, and there may be some loss of dexterity in extremities as the shell/core effect reduces blood flow. Shivering can be mild to severe as the body forces muscles to exercise to generate heat. If fluid volume is not already depleted, cold diuresis will continue, with the patient producing relatively dilute urine.

Vital Signs in Mild Hypothermia

P: Normal

BP: Normal

R: Normal

T: 90–96 degrees Fahrenheit

C: A on AVPU: mild to moderate mental status changes

S: Shell/core effect

Temperatures are best measured rectally, if possible: Shell cooling will cause oral readings to be lower than the core temperature. A special low-reading clinical thermometer is required for measuring core temperature below 94 degrees Fahrenheit.

TREATMENT OF MILD HYPOTHERMIA.

This is an urgent field problem. Unless you can improve heat production and retention, severe hypothermia will soon follow. Field rewarming must be an immediate priority to prevent further problems. Any field rewarming technique is generally safe as long as the patient is awake and able to cooperate with you.

1. Heat Retention. Reduce the cold challenge by sheltering the patient from wind and moisture. Remove wet and cold clothing and redress or wrap the patient in dry insulation, paying special attention to the head and face. A vapor barrier over the clothing, like a plastic or foil blanket, will reduce evaporative cooling and the effect of wind and aid in heat retention. Be sure to insulate from the cold ground with a foam pad or sleeping bag.

Add heat: Build a fire, lay the patient in the sun, or surround him with warm bodies to prevent further cooling. Avoid placing anything hot directly on the skin, because the patient may not be able to feel a developing burn.

2. Heat Production. Produce body heat by providing calories, fluids, and exercise. The fastest way to make calories available for heat production is to feed the patient foods containing lots of simple sugars. This means Twinkies, candy bars, and honey. If you can give sugar in a warm liquid, so much the better, but the sugar itself is more important than the temperature of the food. Simple sugar will be absorbed quickly and burn fast, which is exactly what is needed.

Once the patient has warmed up a bit and his digestive system is working again, fuel stores can be replenished with more complex carbohydrates, fats, and proteins. Now is the time for warmer and less desperate trailside dining with your tofu, whole-grain pancakes, and bacon, which will provide a more steady and long-lasting source of energy. Either that, or send out for a pizza.

This is really just the same concept that you use to start a campfire. First comes the sugar—birch bark and kindling that lights with a match and burns like crazy. Once the heat is available, you add the more complex sources of energy, the sticks and logs. If you're successful, you have a nice, even-burning, nightlong source of heat. Let it die, and you have to start over with the kindling again.

Exercise is an excellent way of warming a well-fed cold person if it can be done without increasing exposure to the cold challenge. Shivering is an involuntary form of exercise that produces a significant amount of heat while burning a lot of calories. Don't try to prevent shivering, just be sure to provide plenty of fuel, and insulation to trap the heat.

SEVERE HYPOTHERMIA

Severe body-core cooling results in a temporary hibernationlike state. The gradual slowing of the circulatory, respiratory, and nervous systems results in a reduced oxygen demand in the tissues at the same time perfusion is being reduced. Life can be preserved for a considerable period of time, but as cooling progresses the major body systems will ultimately fail and death will occur.

It is quite possible to mistake severe hypothermia for death. In the not too distant past, there were many "body recoveries" of lost hikers, hunters, and sailors who probably had vital signs, albeit very faint ones, at the time they were carted off to the morgue. Fortunately, recent advances in the understanding and treatment of severe hypothermia have resulted in completely different field management, and the survival of patients who would otherwise have been given up for dead.

ASSESSMENT OF SEVERE HYPOTHERMIA.

Making the distinction between mild and severe hypothermia is critically important for field treatment. Accurate measurement of core temperature by rectal thermometer can be very helpful when you're trying to decide how to treat, but it is not required.

As the core temperature falls below 90 degrees Fahrenheit, mental status changes will be severe, leading to a decreased consciousness. The severe hypothermic may exhibit bizarre personality changes, hallucinations, and confusion, followed by a drop to V, P, or U on the AVPU scale. He or she will not be able to cooperate with treatment. Shivering will stop as shell cooling and lack of calories to burn deactivates muscles. Cold diuresis may continue if fluid stores are not yet depleted.

Vital Signs in Severe Hypothermia

P: Decreased; may be as slow as one beat per minute

BP: Decreased; may be unobtainable

R: Decreased; may not be observable

T: Below 90 degrees Fahrenheit

C: Severe mental status changes leading to decreased consciousness

S: Cold, pale

Treatment of Severe Hypothermia.

Severely hypothermic patients should be transported as quickly as possible to controlled rewarming in a hospital. Field rewarming is dangerous and should be considered a last resort. During evacuation, the following steps should be taken to stop heat loss:

First, package the patient in dry insulation, ideally on a foam pad in a sleeping bag. Wrap the whole package in a vapor barrier such as a tent fly or ground cloth. Adding heat sources to the insu-

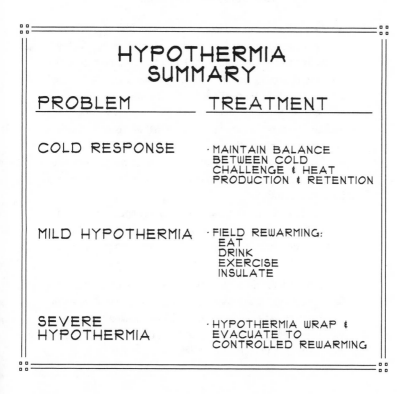

HYPOTHERMIA SUMMARY

PROBLEM	TREATMENT
COLD RESPONSE	· MAINTAIN BALANCE BETWEEN COLD CHALLENGE & HEAT PRODUCTION & RETENTION
MILD HYPOTHERMIA	· FIELD REWARMING: EAT DRINK EXERCISE INSULATE
SEVERE HYPOTHERMIA	· HYPOTHERMIA WRAP & EVACUATE TO CONTROLLED REWARMING

lation layer in the form of chemical heat packs or warmed water bottles will have minimal effect and may not be worth the weight.

Second, transport gently. Because a cold heart muscle is extremely irritable, jostling or other rough handling can cause it to go into ventricular fibrillation. Do not attempt to force exercise. Positive pressure ventilation may be useful if it can be accomplished without endangering the evacuation.

Third, position the patient flat. The blood vessels in the body shell have lost their ability to constrict and will allow blood to escape the core if the patient is held upright. If the patient must be lowered down a cliff or hoisted into a helicopter, do it only with the patient positioned horizontally in a litter. Never allow a vertical hoist!

Case Study—Hypothermia

S: A seventeen-year-old student was removed from the bow of a boat after being on watch without relief for three hours during a cold and wet sail to windward. He had repeatedly been asked if he was cold or would like something to eat and always replied that he was "OK." He responded the same way when asked if he saw anything ahead. Because no one else was particularly excited about replacing him, he remained at his post. Eventually someone noticed that his wool hat had rolled down over his eyes even though he continued to claim to be on lookout. After some debate among the students, this was brought to the instructor's attention.

   The student had no known allergies, was not on medication, had no history of significant medical problems, and his last meal had been over four hours previously. There was no reason to suspect injury.

O: On examination, the student was awake but subdued and confused. He could open his eyes and sit up on command. His foul-weather gear was open in front, and he was soaked to the waist. Vital signs at 16:15 were: BP: 110/70; P: 60; R: 12; C: A on AVPU with lethargy and confusion; T: felt cool; S: pale.

A: Mild Hypothermia

A': Severe Hypothermia

P: Sail was reduced and the boat was turned downwind. One student was detailed to start the stove and another to replace the patient on watch. Other students removed the patient's soaked gear. He was clothed in borrowed polypropylene, placed in a doubled sleeping bag, and wrapped in a plastic tarp. He was assisted in drinking a couple of cups of warm thick cocoa.

Discussion: Although this problem could have been avoided, it was handled appropriately once discovered. The instructor's plan stabilized the scene, reduced the cold challenge, and increased heat retention and production.

This patient showed almost immediate improvement in consciousness and mental status. Evacuation was not initiated, but the instructor chose to continue downwind to an anchorage several miles away. The expedition was continued in the same messy and cold easterly wind the following day, but the entire crew was warm, well fed, and hydrated. Bow watch was rotated regularly.

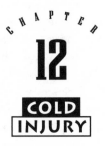

The expansion of water as it turns to ice is an impressive natural phenomenon. Frost action crumbles mountain ranges, cracks engine blocks, and heaves roads. When freezing occurs in your fingers and toes, the effects are no less impressive.

Anything that restricts the circulation of warm blood to tissues allows freezing to occur more readily. For example, getting chilled in cold weather means that the shell/core effect reduces perfusion to the extremities to maintain core temperature. Constricting clothing such as ski boots or a splint tied too tightly can reduce blood flow as well. Cigarette smoking is an additional inhibitor, infusing the body tissues with nicotine, a powerful vasoconstrictor.

I remain forever amazed by the sight of a lightly dressed skier, huddled on the chairlift with the temperature below zero, having his morning cigarette. He should just take off all of his clothes, jump in the snow, and get it over with! Few such people seem to see what skiing hatless and smoking has to do with frostbitten toes. They usually blame their ski boots.

This is not such a big deal at a ski resort with lodges at top and bottom. But in the backcountry, dealing with frostbite is inconvenient at best, and often disastrous. It must be taken seriously both in prevention and in cure.

Certainly, well-insulated and proper-fitting boots, gloves, and face mask can go a long way toward preventing frostbite in extreme conditions. But equally important is maintaining an active and warm body core that will ensure a good supply of warm blood to the extremities. That's why you eat a good breakfast and wear a hat to keep your feet warm.

Sometime when you're not paying attention, or when you are a little hypothermic and not thinking clearly enough to prevent it, tissue will begin to freeze. You won't feel it happening because nerve tissue is the most sensitive to oxygen deprivation and the affected part goes numb when the circulation stops. Ice crystals form in the tissue, doing the same kind of damage ice can do anywhere.

The very early stage of freezing is called frostnip. This occurs when there is a loss of local tissue perfusion with the beginning of ice crystal formation. Only the outer layers of skin are affected, and prompt rewarming at this stage usually causes no disability or tissue loss.

Severe damage, however, can result from prolonged or very deep freezing. Much of the damage occurs during and after rewarming because tissue is very sensitive at this time to further injury, even from normal use. Refreezing is devastating. For a good example of the potential for damage, freeze and thaw a ripe tomato a couple of times. You'll be left with a pile of red mush.

ASSESSMENT OF COLD INJURY

Frostnip is the loss of circulation due to early freezing of the superficial layers of the skin. The area will appear white or gray (pink or red in dark-skinned people) and will feel cold and stiff to the touch. Nevertheless, the area will remain pliable enough to allow movement over unfrozen deeper layers, joints, and tendons. The typical discomfort of early cooling will be replaced by numbness.

Frostnip responds rapidly to rewarming. There will be pain during treatment, with only mild inflammation following. The rewarmed skin will be mildly tender, red, and slightly swollen.

Blistering does not occur. No specific long-term care is required, although the skin will be more susceptible to further cold injury.

Frostbite occurs when the skin and underlying tissues are frozen solid. The area is white or bluish and firm to the touch. Skin does not move over joints or underlying tissues. Ice crystals are usually visible on the skin surface. There is a complete loss of sensation. The digit or extremity feels like a club.

Rewarming is extremely painful and can cause further damage if not done properly. The rewarmed tissues do not look or feel normal. There will be signs of mild to severe inflammation with blisters, swelling, redness, and possible tissue death, which will appear dark blue or black.

Treatment of Cold Injury

Areas of frostnip should be immediately warmed at the first sign of numbness. Left frozen, frostnip can easily progress to frostbite. Like early hypothermia, frostnip is a case for stopping whatever you're doing and making the time and effort to warm up. Usually, just protecting the area from the weather will do it. But remember to reverse the shell/core effect by warming the whole body as well as the affected part. Put a hat on, eat something, and exercise to produce heat. The people who get into trouble with frostbite are the ones who ignore the first signs of frostnip.

Frostbite is best treated by rewarming under controlled conditions. The chances of further damage from trauma and infection are high. Pain will be severe. Usually this means the patient should be in a medical facility. Allowing tissue to remain frozen for several hours during an evacuation is better than uncontrolled field rewarming. This is especially true of frozen feet and hands, which will be impossible to use once rewarmed (remember the tomato).

However, if you find yourself stuck somewhere that makes early evacuation impossible, field rewarming may be your only option. Set up a secure shelter and be sure your patient is warm, dry, well fed, and hydrated. Premedicate with an anti-inflammatory drug like ibuprofen (800 milligrams) taken orally, which will reduce pain and inflammation, and help prevent blood clots from forming in the injured tissue.

Immerse the frozen extremity in water that is 105 degrees Fahrenheit. If you don't have a thermometer, the water should feel hot but not uncomfortable to normal skin. Keep adding warm water to the pot to keep the temperature up as the thawing process continues.

Once the part is rewarmed, it is vital to protect it from trauma. This means no use of the digit or extremity, and absolutely never allow it to refreeze.

Consider rewarmed frostbite to be a high-risk wound. Bandages and splinting are required. Rewarmed frostbite on the feet usually means an air-evacuation or carry-out evacuation if there is no other option.

Frequently monitor distal circulation, sensation, and movement to ensure that splints or bandages do not constrict circulation as swelling develops. If possible, keep the part elevated. Continue regular doses of ibuprofen, and if you have it, cover the area with aloe vera gel or ointment, which has been shown to have both anti-inflammatory and antibacterial properties. Early medical follow-up is essential.

Frostbite that rewarms spontaneously should be protected in the same way. Do not try to prevent rewarming by packing an extremity in snow. If it starts to thaw, stop where you are and tend to it.

TRENCH FOOT

Trench foot is an injury that develops with prolonged exposure to cold and wet conditions above freezing. It is not limited to feet and often involves the hands of paddlers, fishers, and Outward Bound students. Numbness is common due to decreased circulation (perfusion). It does not indicate frostbite, but tissue damage can occur if the conditions persist over days or weeks. Trench foot can also be caused by wearing vapor-barrier boots in cold conditions, which means that high-altitude climbers and sailors or fishermen at sea in cold weather are set up for trench foot.

ASSESSMENT OF TRENCH FOOT

The key is usually the patient's history. The signs and symptoms are typical of a general inflammatory response, with pain, redness, and sometimes blisters. Because the skin's protective barrier is breaking down, bacterial infection can develop, which can really complicate the problem.

TREATMENT OF TRENCH FOOT

If the cause is wet and cold conditions, common sense would suggest that the treatment is warm and dry. As in frostbite, healing tissue can be damaged by further use, so bandaging for protection may be required. Treat any open wounds to prevent infection and allowing healing.

Prevention is worth the trouble. In "trench" conditions, try to give your hands and feet several dry and warm hours each day. Sleep with your wet socks in your sleeping bag to dry them, but not with them on your feet. Take your wet-suit booties and gloves off whenever possible. And when you are wearing waterproof boots, change your socks frequently to keep your feet as dry as you can.

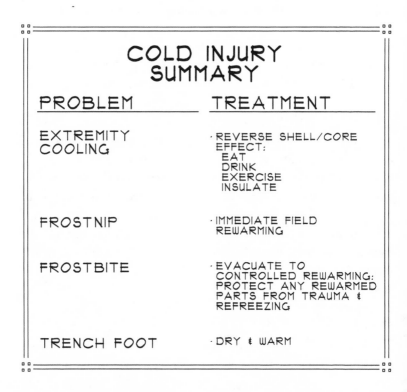

COLD INJURY SUMMARY

PROBLEM	TREATMENT
EXTREMITY COOLING	· REVERSE SHELL/CORE EFFECT: EAT DRINK EXERCISE INSULATE
FROSTNIP	· IMMEDIATE FIELD REWARMING
FROSTBITE	· EVACUATE TO CONTROLLED REWARMING: PROTECT ANY REWARMED PARTS FROM TRAUMA & REFREEZING
TRENCH FOOT	· DRY & WARM

NEAR DROWNING

Drowning is death by respiratory failure because some liquid, usually water, replaces the air in the lungs. This event is most commonly preceded by a loss of muscular coordination due to the rapid shell cooling that occurs in cold-water immersion. No longer able to swim, the patient sinks below the surface and inhales part of the lake, ocean, or river in which she or he is submerged. Even the strongest swimmer can drown this way.

Drowning can also happen almost instantly with the involuntary gasp that sometimes comes with the surprise of sudden immersion. This can affect kayakers rolled by a wave, or fishermen pulled out of the boat by their pot warp or nets. They are immediately deprived of any reserve air and will not remain conscious for more than a few seconds. Most of the time, water fills the lungs all the way to the alveoli. In about 15 percent of the cases, the larynx goes into spasm, closing off the lungs and resulting in a "dry drowning."

A water-filled respiratory system, however, is not always fatal. Sometimes "near drowning," indicating at least temporary survival of water inhalation, occurs in very cold water where the rapid onset of hypothermia offers temporary protection to the brain deprived of oxygen. In rare cases, patients have been resuscitated after spending up to an hour under cold water, with little or no brain damage. What is meant by "cold" is a matter of some debate. Generally, though, any water below about 70 degrees Fahrenheit can be considered cold enough to have the desired effect. The degree of protection offered by the onset of hypothermia increases considerably as water temperature goes down.

ASSESSMENT OF NEAR DROWNING

This is an Initial Assessment problem. You should try to determine how long the patient was submerged, how cold the water is, and how soon Advanced Life Support can be reached. Resuscitation should be attempted if the patient has been under water for less than an hour.

TREATMENT OF NEAR DROWNING

Respiratory failure is treated immediately with positive pressure ventilation. There is no need to drain water from the lungs, and there is no difference in field treatment between salt and fresh water. Confirmed cardiac arrest is treated with CPR.

With hypothermia, the pulse can be very slow and difficult to find. While continuing to perform ventilation, you can allow up to two minutes for the detection of a pulse before beginning chest compressions. This reduces the chance of doing compressions unnecessarily and damaging a still-functioning heart.

Most of the people who have survived drowning were not in cardiac arrest and began breathing on their own within the first two minutes of being taken from the water. Even though they may appear to be much better immediately after rescue, they should be quickly evacuated to medical care. Water is an irritant to lung tissue and will cause the later development of pulmonary fluid. In effect, the patient will begin to drown again as the lungs fill up with water from inside the body.

Those who are in cardiac arrest when they are pulled from the water have a much lower survival rate. In the urban setting, Basic Life Support with cardiopulmonary resuscitation begins immediately. Rapid transport to a hospital with well-controlled resuscitation and rewarming follows close behind. There have been a few dramatic saves made this way.

In the wilderness environment, the survival rate for patients who do not respond quickly to Basic Life Support is about zero. The question of further treatment is controversial. Some authorities suggest that these patients should be treated as severe hypothermics, packaged to prevent heat loss, and transported gently to controlled rewarming in a hospital. However, with the chances for success limited, a dangerous rescue effort may not be justified.

C H A P T E R

14

PROBLEMS
WITH HIGH ALTITUDE

The higher you go in the atmosphere, the less oxygen there is. At about 18,000 feet above sea level, air pressure (hence, air that is available to breath) is reduced by 50 percent. This is accentuated at higher latitudes because the earth's atmosphere is thicker at the equator and thinner at the poles. For example, the effects of altitude on the summit of Denali in Alaska are about 15 percent greater than at the same altitude in the Himalayas.

At a constant altitude, the amount of oxygen in the air does not fluctuate significantly with the temperature, time of day, season, or any other routine environmental changes. No matter where you are, your major body systems will become acclimatized to the location. Your rate of respiration, the number of red blood cells in your circulatory system, and other physiologic processes reach a balance with your environment whether you're a Maine lobsterman or a mountain guide in the Andes.

There are compensatory mechanisms that allow you to change altitude, within limits, without getting out of balance. You can move from sea level to about 8,000 feet with minimal effect. In the short term there will be an increase in respiratory rate to make up for the reduced oxygen. And because you are breathing faster you will blow off more carbon dioxide than usual, causing your blood to become more basic (with an elevated pH). But if you stay at altitude for several days, your kidneys will rebalance the pH of your blood, calibrating your system to the new environment.

If you were to continue to go even higher, your body would compensate and rebalance again. Over the course of weeks you would undergo further physiologic changes, such as producing more red blood cells. Ultimately you would reach the limit of your body's ability to compensate.

This ability of your body to adapt to altitude, and the speed with which it happens, varies widely from person to person. Women seem to be less susceptible to respiratory problems in high altitudes, but otherwise there appears to be no relationship to physical fitness or gender—some people simply adapt to altitude better than others do. However, everyone's ability to adapt to higher altitudes is reduced by alcohol and other depressant drugs, which reduce the nervous system's respiratory drive. Overexertion at the new altitude also inhibits acclimatization.

The best way to adapt to higher altitude is to take your time, stay away from depressants, and take it easy. Allow your normal compensatory mechanisms the time to work by ascending in stages. Climb no faster than your body can adapt. Do not overexert on the first day at the new altitude, and plan to remain there for two to three days before proceeding higher. If you pay attention to what your body is telling you, you should be able to avoid more serious problems.

Push yourself too hard and too fast at extreme altitudes, however, and you can find yourself in big trouble. Severe problems develop when the reduced oxygenation results in capillary leakage and body-tissue swelling. The organs most seriously affected by this are the brain and lungs, resulting in the medical conditions we call high altitude pulmonary edema (HAPE), and high altitude cerebral edema (HACE). The generic problems, of course, are the familiar elevated intracranial pressure (ICP) and pulmonary fluid.

HACE causes the symptoms of what is commonly known as acute mountain sickness. Probably everyone who travels to altitude experiences some degree of brain swelling and elevated ICP, with its associated mild symptoms. But when HACE progresses far enough to significantly increase ICP, more serious symptoms appear. The exact mechanism for this capillary leakage of fluid into the brain is still unknown.

ASSESSMENT AND TREATMENT OF HACE

Mild HACE (or acute mountain sickness) is characterized by mild headache that is easily relieved by aspirin or ibuprofen and slight nausea with little or no vomiting. The patient may experience slight dizziness, loss of appetite, mild fatigue, and some degree of insomnia. This is where two days of prevention is worth 4,000 feet of cure.

The key to prevention is to recognize this mild form of altitude sickness and allow your body time to adapt before climbing any higher. You should avoid sedatives like alcohol or narcotic drugs, which can depress respiration. A drug called Diamox, available by prescription, can be used to increase the rate of respiration by changing blood pH. Taking 125 milligrams twice a day is usually sufficient (please consult a medical practitioner).

Moderate HACE produces severe headaches not relieved by aspirin or ibuprofen, persistent vomiting, and fatigue, typical symptoms of increased ICP. This is treated with pain medication, rest and an immediate descent of 1,000 to 2,000 feet, if possible. The patient should be observed closely for increasing severity of symptoms. Be prepared for an emergency descent if his condition worsens. Supplemental oxygen will be helpful. For a short time, steroid drugs can be used to reduce swelling. A therapeutic dose of Decadron is 4 milligrams every six hours (again, please consult a medical practitioner).

Severe HACE is a life-threatening emergency. The key feature is ataxia (inability to walk straight). The patient will show changes in consciousness and mental status from the very subtle to the very bizarre. The symptoms of severe HACE can be confused or mixed with those of hypoglycemia (low blood sugar), dehydration, hypothermia, hyperthermia, and exercise exhaustion because all can cause a decrease in muscular performance and efficiency as well as changes in consciousness and mental status. Under most field conditions the most practical approach is to target all five problems as possible causes until proven otherwise.

Severe HACE is treated using all the techniques for the mild and moderate forms, plus an immediate descent of 2,000 to 4,000 feet. Exertion should be minimized, but there should be no delay in descent.

A portable device call a Gamow Bag can be used to temporarily increase the air pressure around the patient by about two pounds per square inch, simulating a descent of 5,000 to 6,000 feet. This may substantially improve the patient's condition to the point that he or she can be released from the bag and allowed to walk down before debilitating symptoms reoccur.

ASSESSMENT AND TREATMENT OF HAPE

High altitude pulmonary edema is caused by the constriction of pulmonary arteries in response to reduced levels of oxygen in combination with increased cardiac output (a stronger heartbeat). The increased pressure forces fluid out of the capillaries and into the alveoli, obstructing air exchange. The primary symptom is shortness of breath.

HAPE will be exacerbated by anything that increases fluid retention, for instance, taking salt tablets. It also may be made worse by the shell/core effect in cold weather.

In the early stages, symptoms of HAPE may be limited to mild shortness of breath during exertion, and an infrequent cough. Severe HAPE will cause shortness of breath even at rest and may produce gurgling respirations and a frequent cough that brings forth white or pink sputum. The patient may be in significant distress and appear cyanotic (blue or pale). A low-grade fever may be present. HAPE can be confused with pneumonia or pulmonary contusion from trauma.

The appearance of any degree of HAPE is a bad sign, because the condition tends to progress from bad to worse. Descent to a lower elevation should be a priority. Unfortunately, exertion will make pulmonary edema worse due to increased cardiac output.

There may be situations where it would be better to remain in place rather than perform a strenuous evacuation. A Gamow Bag may save lives.

If symptoms are severe, the generic treatment for respiratory distress should be applied. Supplemental oxygen is helpful temporarily. Diamox seems to be useful only in the early stages of HAPE. If a descent of 2,000 feet does not improve symptoms, another cause for the problem (pneumonia in particular) should be considered.

ALTITUDE PROBLEMS SUMMARY

PROBLEM	TREATMENT
MILD SYMPTOMS OF HACE	· REST UNTIL ADAPTED · PAIN MEDICATION · DIAMOX
MODERATE SYMPTOMS OF HACE	· PAIN MEDICATION · DIAMOX · CONSIDER DESCENT OF 1,000 – 2,000 FEET
SEVERE SYMPTOMS OF HACE OR ANY EVIDENCE OF HAPE	· IMMEDIATE DESCENT OF 2,000 – 4,000 FEET

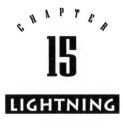

CHAPTER 15

LIGHTNING

I n the heart of a thunderstorm thousands of feet above an air base in eastern Ontario, the friction between violent air currents and particles of water and ice created an enormous negative electrostatic charge. Leader strokes probed toward the positively charged earth and were met a hundred feet above the ground by a pilot stroke probing upward from an air force jet parked on the apron. The newly established pathway became the conductor for a massive discharge of electrical current in a dazzling display of the natural phenomenon we call lightning. Traveling through a channel of ionized air only about an inch in diameter, the current generated 15 million volts at 20,000 amperes in only a thousandth of a second. The shock wave created by the explosive expansion of heated air rolled into the late afternoon as the familiar sound we call thunder. The three air crewmen hiding from the rain under the jet's wing never knew what hit them. They became part of the lightning pathway in an all-too-common example of what we like to call "bad luck."

The most seriously injured man was found twenty feet from the aircraft. The only thing left of his clothing were his boots and necktie, and his heartbeat and breathing had stopped. He had a small burn on his chest where his dog tags had been resting. Only quick action by a Saint John ambulance crew saved the man's life. Even though lightning can be capricious and unpredictable, there are some relatively safe places in which to shelter from a thunderstorm. Standing between a large metal object and the ground is not one of them.

Lightning is the number one weather-related killer in the United States, and it remains an occasional threat as far north as Arctic Canada. You *do* have a better chance of being struck by lightning than by drowning in a flood, being buried in an avalanche, or being sucked out of Kansas by a tornado. In the United States, 800 to 1,000 people are injured by lightning each year, and up to 250 are killed. The highest incidence of activity occurs in New Mexico and Florida.

Lightning is nature's way of equalizing the massive static electric charges that build up between the atmosphere and the ground during violent weather. The actual strike occurs when these charges develop enough potential to overcome atmospheric resistance. The electrical discharge generates millions of volts and tens of thousands of amperes—enough power, you would think, to utterly destroy anything in its path. But this is not always the case.

Only 20 percent of lightning victims die of their injuries. This is probably because, in spite of its massive power, lightning is extremely brief in duration. The average discharge lasts for only about one thousandth of a second, not enough time for much of the electrical energy to overcome skin resistance and enter the body. Most of the current passes over the skin surface on its way to the ground. As a result, the types of internal injuries typical of household current electrocution are rarely seen with lightning.

The energy in lightning is dissipated in the form of heat and light. The instantaneous heating and expansion of the column of air through which the current passes generates the shock wave we hear as thunder. As with any explosion, if a person is close enough to it the shock wave can burst eardrums, break bones, and rupture internal organs.

The direct-current flow in a lightning strike can disrupt the electrochemical function of the nervous system, causing respiratory

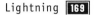

and cardiac arrest. As the current flows over the skin it heats the moisture on the surface, causing superficial burns, and in some cases can generate enough explosive force to tear clothing apart.

The current from lightning can affect you through direct contact if you're really unlucky, or indirectly in the form of ground current or "splash-over." From the point of contact, ground current spreads out through earth, rock, or water and can zap you if you become part of its path. Splash-over can best be described as a much less powerful splinter of the main airborne bolt. Because the energy is diffused, both forms of indirect exposure are generally less devastating than a direct hit.

The extent of injury from current is related to the path the current takes over and through the body. If you're holding onto a steel shroud when the bolt hits your mast, the current may pass through your arm, into your chest, and out your feet. The vital organs of the major body systems can become part of the path, producing life-threatening problems. On the other hand, ground current usually passes onto one foot and off the other, leaving the vital organs outside the path.

Livestock have a particularly bad time with ground current. Because they stand on four legs, often on wet ground, and seldom wear sneakers, the path of current inevitably passes through their chests. Livestock are killed by lightning much more often than people are.

ASSESSMENT OF LIGHTNING INJURY

The Scene Size-up for dangers is particularly important here. Lightning does strike twice, actually many times, in the same place. If the storm is continuing, it may be very dangerous to approach the scene, especially if it is on a hilltop or cliff face. Look for more than one patient; about 30 percent of lightning fatalities involve two or more people.

Although it is rare, the explosive force in a direct strike or near miss can cause all of the injuries typical of massive blunt trauma, including ruptured organs and broken bones. Burns caused by lightning are generally superficial, with more serious deep burns occurring in less than 5 percent of patients. Nervous system disruption is common with many patients experiencing loss of consciousness, and most experience some degree of amnesia (loss of memory). The most common fatal event is cardiac and respiratory arrest.

TREATMENT OF LIGHTNING INJURY

A heart arrested by lightning will often restart on its own, but arrested breathing might need more help. In such cases, the prompt initiation of CPR or positive pressure ventilation can be life saving.

The burns caused by lightning tend to be superficial, but the associated fluid loss can cause shock and hypothermia. In any large-area burn, intravenous fluids and protection from heat loss are important. Shock, anticipated shock, head injury and ICP, and musculoskeletal trauma should all be treated as you would do with any other patient. The evacuation of a lightning-strike patient is important, even if he or she is stabilized, because heart and nervous system problems can develop hours or days later.

PREVENTION OF LIGHTNING INJURY

Lightning is pretty much going to go where it wants so the trick is to avoid being there at the same time. You know the obvious: Stay off hilltops, ridges, and open water, and generally try to avoid being the highest thing around. You also don't want to be in contact with an isolated tree or other likely target.

In the field, the best tactic is to squat with your feet together as low as you can, ideally on your foam pad or backpack, which will help insulate you from ground current. A group should be well spread out, so that a strike will not incapacitate everybody at once. Aboard a larger boat, avoid having the whole crew clustered in the cockpit. Water is a good conductor of electricity, so don't swim or wade during a thunderstorm. Because there is some evidence that wearing metal objects increases the likelihood of injury, remove earrings, metal glasses, backpacks, and anything similar.

Theoretically, there is a safety zone on the ground or water about 45 degrees out from the top of a tall object. How reliable this formula is remains in question, but I like to anchor about 45 degrees

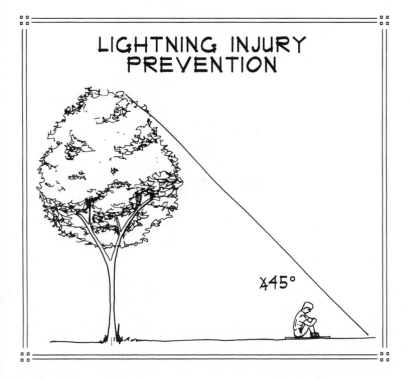

LIGHTNING INJURY
PREVENTION

≯45°

out from the tallest mast in the harbor when lightning is likely, nonetheless, just in case this theory has some credibility.

Another relatively safe place is inside a car. The insulating value of the tires offers protection from ground current, and the metal shell will conduct the energy of a direct strike around the occupants and into the ground. This is why our injured air crewman would have been much better off *inside* the aircraft. The metal shrouds and stays on a sailing vessel may have the same conductive effect, provided there is a path to the water, like a good grounding system or heavy cable led over the side from a shroud.

On a cliff, you're really in a tough spot. Lightning current will follow the cliff face, especially where it's wet, like down your belay line. Hollows and caves may seem attractive, but current can jump across a cave opening and include you in its path. A cave must be about three times as deep as the size of the opening to be safe, and you should be well back from the entrance.

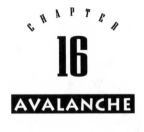

CHAPTER 16

AVALANCHE

Predicting and avoiding avalanches is a topic worthy of its own text. As more people enter the backcountry for recreation, avalanche deaths in the United States are increasing sharply. It is interesting to note that the vast majority of avalanche victims are experienced skiers and mountaineers with some degree of avalanche awareness training.

In avalanche rescue, the most important factor in survival is speed of recovery. In the first fifteen minutes, 86 percent of avalanche victims are found alive. This drops to about 50 percent for the period between fifteen and thirty minutes, and is much lower thereafter. It makes sense that most of the victims that survive are dug out by the people traveling with them, not by rescue teams arriving hours later.

In spite of this grim outlook, no one buried in an avalanche should be given up for dead based on time. A few people have survived very long burials. The record in the United States is twenty-two hours, and there are stories from Europe of people being found alive after days under the snow.

The most common and serious major system problem in avalanche rescue is airway obstruction, either directly because of snow packed into the nose and mouth, or indirectly by burial. Snow is mostly air and often very porous. If the victim can succeed in creating an air space around the face, survival for a short period of time is possible. Eventually, a layer of nonporous ice will form around the victim, cutting off the air supply.

Hypothermia is rarely an immediate problem with the avalanche survivor. The people who get caught in avalanches are usually well dressed for the weather, and snow is a good insulator. Unfortunately, this means that respiratory failure will kill the victim long before any protective effect of severe hypothermia is realized.

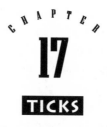

C H A P T E R

17

TICKS

Ticks themselves are not much of a problem. They mind their own business, cause no pain, eat very little, and depart quietly when they're done. Not bad, for a biting arthropod.

But like lots of other creatures, ticks carry disease, including the current favorites Rocky Mountain spotted fever, Colorado tick fever, tick paralysis, and Lyme disease. Most of these diseases produce a constellation of confusing symptoms and are not easy to diagnose. It is much easier to avoid contracting the disease in the first place, and this means avoiding ticks. Experts on the subject recommend wearing a long-sleeved shirt with long pants tucked into high socks, and a hat with an attached bandana that covers the neck. Apply insect repellent to clothing, especially around cuff and neck openings, and on exposed skin. By following these recommendations you will reduce the chances of feeding a tick and acquiring a tickborne disease. You will also, regrettably, sweat bullets, smell like a toxic waste dump, and look twice as scary as the fashion models in the sporting goods catalogs.

Another option is to get into the habit of frequently looking for ticks on your skin and clothing. They usually like to crawl around for a while before settling in to feed, so frequent inspections will increase the chances of getting them before they attach themselves. Attached ticks can be removed by gently prying them off with tweezers. Sometimes the mouth parts will break off and be left in the skin. Try to scrape these out with a sharp blade or

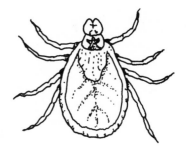

needle. Prompt removal of ticks will help prevent the spread of disease. Lyme disease, for example, is not effectively transmitted until the tick has been in place for a day or so.

The place and time to be vigilant for ticks is in areas of vegetation such as woods, grass, and brush during the spring, summer, and fall. Adult ticks are eight-legged arthropods ranging in size from nearly microscopic to a centimeter in diameter. The ticks of greatest concern are 2–4 millimeters in diameter, which, before they begin to feed, are easily recognized as a foreign creature on your skin. Once attached and engorged with blood, they look more like a wart, mole, or other skin part and may be missed by someone who doesn't know your body as well as you do. The appearance of flulike symptoms, rash, and muscular aches and pains several days to weeks after a confirmed long-term tick attachment is worth bringing to the attention of a medical practitioner.

SECTION VI

Common Symptoms

and

Medical Problems

18

A GENERAL
APPROACH TO ILLNESS

A s a medical practitioner, I much prefer treating trauma to treating illness. Something that is merely broken or torn usually presents a straightforward mechanical problem. Illness, on the other hand, is often confusing and scary and defies a quick fix. The nonspecific symptoms of many illnesses generate a long list of possible diagnoses. In the hospital it can be very difficult to figure out exactly what you're dealing with. In the backcountry, it can be impossible.

There is little value in leafing through lists of symptoms and descriptions of diseases just so you can put a name on your patient's problem. The laboratory and X ray aren't available to confirm your suspicions anyway. Your primary job in dealing with illness is to keep your patient safe, comfortable, well hydrated, and to watch for the development of anything serious. The human body is a remarkable organism and will heal itself just fine in the vast majority of cases.

As you evaluate an illness, beware of focusing too much attention on the numbers. By all means, take vital signs, but don't forget to look at the patient. His or her behavior is more important than statistics. You should worry much more about a confused and lethargic person with a temperature of 99 degrees than an active and ori-ented patient with a fever of 104 degrees.

A healthy person willingly takes in food and fluid and produces urine and feces in more or less proportional amounts. She is inter-ested in her surroundings and knows who she is and what she's doing. She will freely move, dress, and protect herself from the environment.

A patient who is ill but basically OK may be grumpy and uncomfortable but will continue to eat and drink and function more or less normally. You don't need to worry about him too much. It is when your patient stops eating and drinking, loses interest in his surroundings, and is unable to take care of himself that you should consider the situation serious. This is the time to be looking for expert help, regardless of the diagnosis.

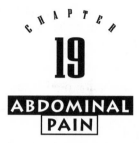

CHAPTER
19

ABDOMINAL
PAIN

The word "abdomen" is a derivation of the Latin word for "hidden," and rightly so. Everything that goes on inside the abdomen is well hidden from our eyes and can become the subject of a lot of conjecture and consternation. How do you know if your crew member's belly pain is resulting from a developing appendicitis or an underdeveloped ability to digest whole grains? Should you call a passing ship for a lift back to Portland or stick it out until you reach Bermuda?

Abdominal pain creates plenty of grief for almost everyone, including experienced surgeons using a variety of diagnostic tests and tools. Even they have a difficult time figuring out what's going on inside a sore abdomen, so don't feel too bad if you can't figure it out either. Focus instead on the *one* important question: Is this pain the symptom of a serious problem?

For our purposes, we can consider the abdomen to be hiding three major components: hollow organs, solid organs, and the sensitive abdominal lining called the peritoneum. Hollow structures, like the stomach, intestines, and gallbladder, contain digestive fluids and have muscular walls that contract rhythmically to move these fluids along the digestive system. The ureters and urinary bladder use similar structure and function to contain and move urine from the kidneys to the outside.

Solid organs have a variety of functions and associated diseases, but we worry mostly about their potential for rupture in abdominal trauma. For example, the liver, spleen, and kidneys, part of the body core, can split open like a watermelon dropped from a truck and bleed profusely.

The peritoneum is a membrane that lines all of the organs and the abdominal wall inside the body cavity. It is exquisitely sensitive to irritation from things like blood, bacteria, and digestive fluids that have gotten loose inside the cavity as a result of injury or illness. The peritoneum also represents a large surface area (greater than that of your skin), which, when inflamed, can leak a large volume of fluid in a short period of time.

ASSESSMENT OF ABDOMINAL PAIN

The nerve cells in hollow organs transmit pain sensations primarily when they are stretched, as when you distend your stomach with a big Thanksgiving dinner. The pain of distention gets worse when the organ system attempts its normal rhythmic muscular contractions.

The intermittent stretching of the hollow organs of the digestive system creates an abdominal pain that, though unpleasant, is usually no cause for concern. It is just the result of gas, fluid, and spasm created by a viral illness or food intolerance, or a buildup of stool (constipation). The pain is the generalized crampy type that precedes a bout of diarrhea or flatulence, after which you feel a whole lot better. The problem is well contained within the intestine and, when it's relieved, the system returns to normal.

With hollow-organ pain you will know that real problems are beginning when whatever is happening begins to irritate the peritoneal lining. Unlike hollow-organ pain, peritoneal pain is location-specific and constant. Movement makes it worse, because the inflamed membrane rubs against itself.

In the classic case of appendicitis, for example, the problem begins with the obstruction of the appendix, which is a part of the hollow intestine in the lower right quadrant of the abdomen. This obstruction leads to infection and swelling. The early symptoms are often the generalized crampy discomfort typical of intestinal distention, and you would probably not label it as serious. But as the infection develops, the swollen and inflamed appendix will begin to irritate the peritoneal lining of the intestine and abdomen. The symptoms will begin to change from generalized cramping to localized constant pain in the right lower quadrant. If the condition gets bad enough, the organ will burst, spilling digestive enzymes and pus into the abdominal cavity. At that point, the whole peritoneum becomes inflamed, with swelling and fluid leakage. If you don't have immediate access to a hospital, shock and death are almost inevitable.

The key to early recognition of this serious problem is the change in character of the pain from crampy and generalized to constant and localized. The same is true of other hollow-organ problems like cholecystitis (gallbladder infection), ectopic pregnancy (fetus in the fallopian tube), and bowel obstruction. It is not necessary to know exactly what you're dealing with to know that it needs a surgeon and an operating room.

Solid organs have few nerve endings that sense pain. Most of the discomfort with solid-organ problems comes from irritation of the peritoneal lining due to infection or bleeding. Both are serious. Blunt trauma with a ruptured solid organ can lead to shock, which should be anticipated in cases of persistent abdominal pain following injury. Again, pain tends to be localized and constant.

Another common source of abdominal discomfort following trauma or exertion is pain in the muscles of the abdominal wall. Although this is not associated with any internal organs and is not serious, it can be difficult to distinguish from peritoneal irritation. This type of pain will usually be relieved by rest and made worse by use of the injured muscles.

If abdominal pain is accompanied by vomiting or diarrhea, you need to be thinking about volume shock from dehydration. This is a big killer of young children and older patients, especially with diseases like cholera. In the backcountry, rehydration can be difficult or impossible.

Diagramming and discussing all of the possible causes of abdominal pain would quadruple the size of this book, but it still would not help you much in the backcountry or far out to sea. Even if you could tell an ectopic pregnancy from appendicitis, you're not going to haul out your fillet knife and operate on either one. What you really want to know is: serious or not serious, evacuate or wait and watch? The following red flag symptoms should help in your decision.

Red Flags for Potentially Serious Problems

Persistent fever

Blood by mouth or rectum

Persistent vomiting or diarrhea

Pain that does not get better within twelve hours

Pain that becomes progressively worse and more localized

Severe tenderness on exam

Signs of volume shock

TREATMENT OF ABDOMINAL PAIN

Treat the cause, which usually means getting the patient out of the field. Whether you're a surgeon or a woodcutter, red flags mean evacuation. You should continue to monitor the patient during transport and note any changes in his or her condition. Even though the problem may eventually resolve itself or show itself to be less serious, it's always better to cancel or slow down an evacuation in progress than to start one too late.

Give fluids to make up for normal and abnormal losses. This is best restricted to water and rehydration solutions. We know that surgeons and anesthesiologists would prefer a patient with an empty stomach, but maintaining fluid volume is critical to survival in the long-term-care situation.

Oral pain medication should be restricted to acetaminophen (Tylenol) because other anti-inflammatory drugs can irritate the gut. Injectable pain medication is preferable. See also the related topics of vomiting, diarrhea, constipation, and dehydration in Chapters 4, 23, 21, and 22, respectively.

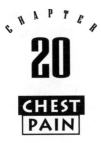

20

CHEST PAIN

J ust about anybody who enters a hospital emergency department
and uses the words "chest" and "pain" in the same sentence gets
evaluated for heart attack (myocardial ischemia or myocardial
infarction). This is almost instinctive, even though medical practitioners know that there are many causes of chest pain that have
nothing to do with the heart. They recognize that the risk and
expense involved in testing for heart attack is much lower than the
risk and expense involved in failing to detect one. For the hospital,
the choice is easy and the policy is clear. Unfortunately, this does
not translate very well to the remote environment, where we need
a much better indication of a real heart problem to balance against
the hazards of evacuation.

ASSESSMENT OF CHEST PAIN

Just as the hospital does, we look for a reasonable explanation for
the pain, and this may include the ischemic heart muscle. More
often, however, it can be attributed to one of a number of other pos-
sibilities. The most common in the backcountry setting is muscle or
rib pain from exercise or injury. This type of pain can usually be

reproduced by movement. There is often a tender area in the same spot where the patient complains of pain. It is usually relieved by rest and aspirin or ibuprofen. The patient does not usually appear otherwise sick, or short of breath.

Chest pain from respiratory infection or lung injury will usually have a pretty clear history of preceding illness. It may be accompanied by cough, fever, and sore throat. It is usually made worse by coughing and deep breathing. The patient is usually somewhat ill in appearance. This pain may be part of a serious respiratory system problem but is not an indication of heart attack.

The pain associated with indigestion is usually accompanied by burping, heartburn, and nausea. Unlike the pain of heart attack, it is often relieved by antacids. The patient will often give a long-standing history of similar episodes associated with certain foods or stress.

The chest pain of a heart attack is caused by ischemia (inadequate perfusion) of the heart muscle due to spasm or clotting in the coronary (heart) arteries. It is typically described as being in the middle of the chest, radiating to the jaw and left arm. The pain is often referred to as "crushing or constricting." There may be shortness of breath and sweating. In a few cases, vital signs will show an irregular heartbeat and the signs of shock (cardiogenic shock). At least this is what the textbook says.

Unfortunately, the classic pattern does not occur in all cases of heart attack. It can be mistaken for indigestion, respiratory infection, or chest-wall pain. In fact, the patient will be trying very hard to mistake it for anything but heart attack. If there is no other obvious cause, we must consider the possibility that the chest pain is due to myocardial ischemia. This is more likely when the patient has some of the risk factors associated with heart disease.

Risk Factors Creating a Higher Risk of Heart Attack

Smoking

Overweight

Sedentary lifestyle

Past history of myocardial ischemia or infarction

History of high blood cholesterol

History of high blood pressure

Male over forty-five years of age

Female after menopause

Family history of heart disease

This does not mean that your slim, nonsmoking, athletic twenty-year-old girlfriend can't have heart problems. It just means that it is very unlikely, and you are not going to call for a heroic evacuation with that thought in mind. But if your chest-pain patient is your overweight, two-pack-a-day smoking fifty-five-year-old law firm partner, you'd best get him out of the woods. This does not mean he *is* having a heart attack, but the likelihood is high enough to justify evacuation.

TREATMENT OF SUSPECTED HEART ATTACK

1. Basic Life Support

2. Rest and reassurance

3. Oxygen if available

4. Evacuation—quick, but not stressful

5. Medication. As long as your patient is not already taking anticoagulant (blood-thinning) medications, give one aspirin tablet with a cup of water. This will reduce the tendency of the blood to clot, which may reduce ischemia in heart muscle. If the patient has other heart medication, such as nitroglycerine, assist him in taking it according to directions.

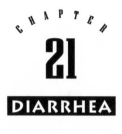

21

DIARRHEA

One of the functions of the large intestine is to absorb fluid from feces just before excretion. This serves to conserve the body's fluid balance and allows you some degree of control over when and where excretion occurs. Diarrhea develops when the lining of the intestinal space is irritated by infection or toxins and fails to absorb fluid. The intestine can, in addition, leak more body fluid on its own, contributing to general fluid loss.

ASSESSMENT OF DIARRHEA

As with abdominal pain, what we want to know is, is it serious or not serious? Diarrhea that is a softer version of normal stool and occurs relatively infrequently in an otherwise healthy individual is usually nothing to worry about. Even if it lasts for several days or weeks, such fluid losses can be replaced by oral intake.

However, diarrhea can be a symptom of other more serious problems, especially when it occurs in the presence of abdominal pain. Diarrhea itself becomes a real problem when fluid loss occurs so rapidly that it cannot be replaced by drinking and eating.

Red Flags for Potentially Serious Problems

Fluid loss in excess of oral replacement volume

Signs of volume shock

Blood in stool

Fever

Persistent pain (see Chapter 19)

TREATMENT OF DIARRHEA

Diarrhea that does not show red flag symptoms can sometimes be helped by bismuth subsalicylate (Pepto-Bismol) or similar over-the-counter preparations. Beware of drugs such as Lomotil, which inhibit intestinal motility, especially in the presence of fever. If the cause of the diarrhea is an intestinal bacterium or parasite, obstructing drainage can increase the severity of the infection.

Most important, you should pay attention to replacing fluid losses with oral intake. Giving water with a pinch of salt and sugar added will replace some body electrolytes. Time will usually correct the situation, but if the problem persists longer than a week, medical advice should be sought.

When red flag signs are noted, evacuation should be considered. If signs of volume shock are present, evacuation should be urgent if fluids cannot be replaced rapidly in the field. During evacuation, give oral fluid as constantly as the patient can tolerate.

CHAPTER

22

CONSTIPATION

Constipation is usually the result of the large intestine doing just what it's supposed to do: absorb fluid from feces. If you are dehydrated, fluid recovery can turn feces into something resembling metamorphic rock and make them tough for even the most energetic hollow-organ muscle contractions to expel.

PREVENTION OF CONSTIPATION

Maintaining fluid balance by staying well hydrated will make it unnecessary for the large intestine to absorb too much fluid from feces. A good indicator for hydration is urine production. You should drink enough fluid to produce light-yellow-colored urine frequently.

Take the time and find the privacy for a decent bowel movement. This is especially difficult on boats at sea in rough conditions or on a big wall climb, when relieving oneself becomes a life-threatening adventure. Nevertheless, it is extremely important. If feces sit in the intestine long enough, solidification will occur no matter how well hydrated you are. Diets high in fiber create bulk that stimulates bowel contraction and holds water in the fecal material.

ASSESSMENT OF CONSTIPATION

We are told by the advertising media that at least one well-formed stool a day is the birthright of every human being. Less than that, and our diet and lifestyle are all wrong. There may be some truth to this, but such a schedule is often unrealistic in the backcountry.

Constipation is annoying when you feel bad because of it, but it becomes a problem when the rest of the body begins to suffer. Exactly when this occurs is highly individual. We have had students go nine days before mentioning they haven't had a bowel movement, whereas others become cranky after only twenty-four hours.

TREATMENT OF CONSTIPATION

Bulk agents like Metamucil and similar substances work like a high-fiber diet. These can be carried in very small gel-capsule form as a dietary supplement.

Osmotic agents like milk of magnesia draw water into the intestine.

Lubricants like mineral oil taken by mouth will smooth intestinal and stool surfaces, moving things along with less effort and pain.

Laxatives, including Ex-Lax and bisacodyl (Dulcolax) suppositories can be used if the treatments above fail. Bisacodyl is generally easier to use because its stimulant effect is limited to the rectum, so it causes less abdominal cramping.

Enemas are generally viewed as a last resort, but they are very safe and effective. Infusing warm water into the rectum (an enema) will hydrate and soften stool, creating the additional bulk necessary to stimulate bowel contraction. Do not use an enema in the presence of red flags for abdominal pain, because the additional pressure may cause hollow-organ rupture.

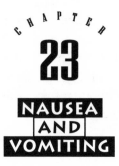

NAUSEA AND VOMITING

L ike diarrhea, vomiting can be the result of a problem with the gastrointestinal system, or it can be a symptom of other problems, such as motion sickness, toxic ingestion, head injury, or infection. Finding and treating the primary cause is the priority. However, you must also consider the additional problems that can be created by the severe fluid loss associated with vomiting.

ASSESSMENT OF VOMITING

Vomiting associated with the following red flags is considered serious. This includes seasickness that is persistent and not responsive to medication, and any persistent vomiting.

Red Flags for Vomiting

Fluid losses cannot be replaced by drinking

Symptoms associated with the red flags for abdominal pain

TREATMENT OF VOMITING

Replace fluid losses as for diarrhea. Give only clear liquids or dilute electrolyte solutions.

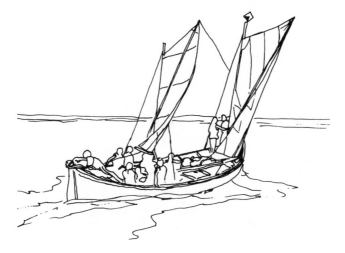

Protect the airway. Vomiting can cause airway obstruction or pulmonary edema if the vomit is inhaled. Position the patient to allow drainage.

Evacuate if red flags are present.

There are many antiemetic drugs. One of the most common and useful is Benadryl (diphenhydramine), which is also used for allergy and cold symptoms. Being able to give drugs by rectal suppository is a real advantage in persistent vomiting. Phenergan or Tigan suppositories might be a good addition to an expedition medical kit. Consult a medical practitioner.

C H A P T E R
24

EAR AND SINUS PROBLEMS

EXTERNAL EAR INFECTION (SWIMMER'S EAR)

Swimmer's ear is an inflammation of the external auditory canal, the tube leading from the outside environment to the outside surface of the eardrum. The problem is usually caused by bacteria that invade skin that is softened by prolonged contact with water.

ASSESSMENT OF SWIMMER'S EAR

As with any infection, swimmer's ear will be characterized by redness, warmth, swelling, and pain. The external structures of the ear and surrounding area will be tender to touch, and the ear canal itself will be extremely sensitive. There is usually a history of recent and repetitive immersion in water.

TREATMENT OF SWIMMER'S EAR

The treatment of choice is antibiotic ear drops, available by a physician's prescription. In lieu of that, regular cleansing of the ear canal with rubbing alcohol followed by mineral oil should reduce the amount of debris and bacteria and contribute to healing. Do not use dry cotton swabs because they will further irritate the ear canal.

Staying out of the water and allowing the ear to heal will help considerably.

MIDDLE EAR INFECTION AND SINUSITIS

The area referred to as the middle ear begins inside the eardrum and extends through a narrow opening into the nasal cavity. It is similar in structure to the other sinuses, which are open spaces lined by mucous membranes with narrow openings into the nose. Middle ear infection and sinusitis are good examples of obstruction and infection. The usual cause is swelling and inflammation from a viral infection or from exposure to water when swimming. The obstructed space fills with fluid, which becomes colonized by bacteria.

ASSESSMENT OF SINUSITIS

The typical sign of sinus infection is facial or ear pain. There will often be a history of several days of mild cold or flu symptoms with a stuffy or runny nose. Bending over at the waist increases pressure in the affected sinus or ear and increases the pain. Sinusitis in the form of middle ear infection can be differentiated from swimmer's ear by the fact that, in sinusitis, although the ear hurts, the external ear structures and ear canal are not red, swollen, or tender to touch. In more severe infections, you may see some discharge of green or yellow pus from the nose or from the ear if the eardrum ruptures. Fever is another symptom of serious infection.

TREATMENT OF SINUSITIS

Sinusitis can be improved by drainage. A middle ear infection may drain spontaneously through a weak point in the eardrum, which is actually a natural protective mechanism. If pain is relieved and no fever develops, there is no emergency in this. Keep the ear dry and see your doctor when you get ashore.

Otherwise, we can try to reduce the swelling of the narrow sinus openings by using decongestant nasal spray or having the patient breathe the steam from a pot of hot water. Systemic decongestants such as Sudafed tablets, or antihistamines like Benadryl will also help. It is important to keep your patient well hydrated, which will keep mucus from drying and becoming too thick to drain. Antibiotics are often necessary for complete treatment if the infection is well established.

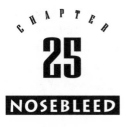

CHAPTER

25

NOSEBLEED

It doesn't take much trauma to rupture the blood vessels in the nose. The most easily injured ones are near the front of the nose (anterior) where bleeding will drain out of the nose if the patient is positioned upright with the head held forward.

ASSESSMENT OF NOSEBLEED

The task here is to distinguish a simple nosebleed from something more significant. If the bleeding started spontaneously, or after blowing or picking the nose, you can be pretty sure it's not complicated. However, if the bleed is the result of trauma, you must consider the possibility of facial-bone fracture and head injury.

TREATMENT OF NOSEBLEED

First, calm your patient and have her sit down. Position her to allow for drainage out of the nose, and have her gently blow out any clots. This sounds scary, but it won't cause the bleeding to get worse. Now, you or the patient should pinch her nostrils together and hold firmly for *fifteen minutes* while she remains sitting upright. This applies simple direct pressure to the most likely source of bleeding.

Remember, to stop the bleeding, it is essential to hold enough pressure for a long enough time. This should stop most of the nosebleeds you are likely to see.

If you encounter a persistent bleed in the field, your best response is the same as for any other bleeding you are unable to control: Make the patient comfortable and prepare for an evacuation. If the patient needs to lie down, protect the airway by positioning her face-down or on her side, with her chest and head supported to allow for drainage from the nose and mouth. A carry-out evacuation may be necessary if volume shock develops.

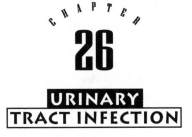

26

URINARY
TRACT INFECTION

U rinary tract infection is most common in women because it is fairly easy for normal skin-surface or intestinal bacteria to migrate from the outside into the normally sterile bladder, where they can reproduce rapidly and begin to invade and inflame the bladder's soft-tissue lining. Normally, frequent urination flushes bacteria out of the bladder and urethra, preventing this from happening.

In both the civilized and backcountry settings there are a number of ways this system can be upset. Perhaps the most common to the wilderness traveler is urinary retention, usually due to slight dehydration. The body's normal efforts to preserve fluid results in low urine output and infrequent flushing of the urinary tract. The same situation can occur simply through lack of opportunity to urinate, such as when one "holds it" until morning rather that getting out of a warm sleeping bag in the middle of the night. Either way, any bacteria entering the bladder and urethra have a longer period of time in which to multiply and invade the tissue lining.

Another common cause of urinary tract infection in females is inadequate hygiene. In settings where bathing is difficult or impossible, the number of bacteria on the outer surface of the skin increases dramatically. Add this to the habit of "drip drying" instead of using toilet paper and you have a greater opportunity for infection.

A third mechanism for infection is direct trauma to the urethra. The usual culprit is frequent or vigorous sexual activity, but it can also be caused by the saddle of a mountain bike, or a climbing harness. This is the so-called honeymoon cystitis, where the urethral opening becomes inflamed, is invaded by bacteria, and becomes infected.

More complicated and dangerous infections can develop when the bacteria climb beyond the bladder to invade the ureters and kidneys. Any sexually transmitted disease is also considered more dangerous because the bacterium or virus is foreign to the body and is more difficult to eradicate. *In males, infection of the urinary tract is unusual because the urethra is so much longer than it is in females, and such infection always indicates a complicated condition. The most common cause is sexually transmitted disease.*

ASSESSMENT OF URINARY TRACT INFECTION

The classic symptoms of uncomplicated urinary tract infection include low pelvic pain; frequent urination in small amounts; cloudy or blood-tinged urine; and pain, tingling, or burning on urination.

In the female, it is possible to confuse infection of the urinary tract with vaginal infection. Inflammation of the vagina and external genitalia can also cause pain and burning on urination (see Chapter 27).

Symptoms that indicate infection has progressed beyond the superficial lining of the urethra and bladder can include any of those just outlined plus the following red flags:

> **Red Flags in Urinary Tract Infection That Indicate a Serious Problem**
>
> Fever
>
> Back pain and tenderness (kidney involvement)
>
> Urinary tract infection in the male
>
> Sexually transmitted disease

TREATMENT OF URINARY TRACT INFECTION

Symptoms of urinary tract infection accompanied by red flags indicate a possibly serious problem, especially if it involves infection of the kidneys, which can become a life-threatening condition treatable only with antibiotics.

The treatment for uncomplicated urinary tract infection usually includes the use of antibiotics as well. Temporary measures, pending access to medical care, involve treating urinary tract infection like any other soft-tissue infection, with drainage and cleansing. Keep the external genitalia as clean as possible and drink plenty of fluids to irrigate the infection.

One nonprescription treatment that can sometimes eradicate an uncomplicated infection is vitamin C taken orally: 1 gram four times a day. Vitamin C is an acid (ascorbic acid), and only a small amount can be absorbed by the body at a time. The excess is excreted in the urine, making it too acidic to harbor most strains of bacteria. One day of treatment with high-dose vitamin C may be enough.

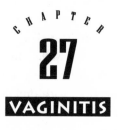

27

VAGINITIS

I nflammation and infection of the vagina often occur when something upsets the normal ecological balance between yeast and bacteria, allowing one of the species to grow out of control. For example, taking penicillin for a strep throat will kill many of the bacteria in the vagina. This opens the way for an overgrowth of yeast, which is not affected by penicillin. Changes in the vaginal environment caused by clothing, sexual activity, stress, and other factors can upset this balance as well.

ASSESSMENT OF VAGINITIS

Vaginitis typically causes itching or burning, and a whitish vaginal discharge sometimes described as "cheesy." There may also be tingling or burning as urine irritates inflamed tissues, causing some confusion with urinary tract infection.

Vaginitis can become dangerous when it begins to spread to other organs. Bacteria can migrate into the uterus and fallopian tubes, causing the infection known as pelvic inflammatory disease. The symptoms will include the easily recognized red flags for abdominal pain.

TREATMENT OF VAGINITIS

Needless to say, suspected pelvic inflammatory disease warrants evacuation to medical care. Simple vaginitis may respond to nonprescription treatment in the field. A temporary reduction of symptoms, or even a complete cure, can be achieved by a douche that is made by diluting a teaspoon of Povidone iodine solution in a quart of water and used once a day for several days. An alternative douche solution may be prepared by adding one tablespoon of vinegar to one quart of water. Douches should not be used by pregnant patients.

Nonprescription medications like Lotrimin cream or suppositories are available for common yeast infections. The manufacturers warn against relying on these treatments unless the patient is fairly certain of the diagnosis through past experience. Because yeast and bacteria grow well in a warm and moist environment, the situation can also be improved by staying dry and cool. This means wearing loose-fitting clothing and spending less time in a wet suit.

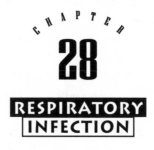

C H A P T E R

28

RESPIRATORY INFECTION

The common cold, with its stuffy nose, sore throat, runny eyes, and cough, has plagued people for eons. There is no reason to believe that it won't pick on you, expedition or no expedition. You should be ready to deal with it.

The mild respiratory infections that we label "colds" or "flu" are caused by viruses. They produce a multiplicity of symptoms that conspire to keep us miserable until our body's immune system identifies the bug, produces specific antibodies, and eradicates it. Problems develop when the virus is particularly virulent, or when the viral infection opens the way for a secondary bacterial infection to take hold. This is how people who start with a cold can end up with a bacterial pneumonia, bronchitis, or strep throat.

ASSESSMENT OF UPPER-RESPIRATORY INFECTION

Mild upper-respiratory infection is characterized by runny nose, mild headache, sneezing, coughing, tearing eyes, mild sore throat, muscular aches, and intermittent fever. Other than being annoyed and uncomfortable, the patient is usually not significantly impaired in her ability to perform normal tasks.

More serious respiratory disease may evolve from the above symptoms or progress independently. Coughing typically becomes productive of thick yellow, green, or brown sputum, a development otherwise known as "coughing in colors." The patient may experience chills, shortness of breath, and chest pain on respiration. Fever will be more persistent.

TREATMENT OF UPPER-RESPIRATORY INFECTION

The treatment of mild upper-respiratory infection involves making the patient more comfortable while her body works to defeat the virus. Use whatever over-the-counter medications make the patient feel better while not interfering with her ability to function. Local decongestants such as nasal sprays, systemic decongestants, and non-narcotic cough medications are very helpful. So is anti-inflammatory medication like ibuprofen.

Equally important is maintaining fluid balance, eating well, staying warm, and getting enough rest. This reduces the number of stressors that the body has to deal with. The system will then be free to focus on fighting the virus and preventing a secondary bacterial invasion.

The patient who is coughing in colors usually needs antibiotics. If you are equipped with these drugs and know which ones to use, the patient can safely be treated in the field if he is otherwise OK. But the availability of antibiotics should not cause you to delay the evacuation of a patient in respiratory distress.

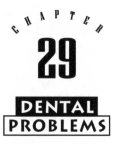

29

DENTAL PROBLEMS

Teeth become a problem when they are fractured or avulsed (knocked out) by trauma and become a nightmare when infected. Not only is there pain, but the pain can interfere with eating and drinking, which is essential to survival. Anyone planning an extended wilderness trip or ocean passage should have any potential problems checked by a dentist before departure.

ASSESSMENT OF DENTAL TRAUMA

Assessment of dental trauma is directed at ensuring that potential major body system problems are considered and stabilized. Immediately make sure that loose teeth, or pieces of teeth, are not obstructing the airway. Other potential dangers to consider are that damage to teeth can be associated with head and neck injury, pain can produce Acute Stress Reaction, and swallowing blood can cause vomiting. Beyond an association with major body system dangers, broken teeth do not represent a medical emergency.

TREATMENT OF DENTAL TRAUMA

First, remove avulsed or fractured teeth that might obstruct the airway. While protecting the cervical spine, position the patient to allow drainage of blood and debris out of the mouth, rather than down the throat.

If the patient is awake and cooperative, have him rinse his mouth with cool water. This will clean out blood clots and loose teeth and help to stop bleeding. Examine the mouth with a flashlight. Look for teeth that are loose or fractured but still in the sockets. Look for empty sockets that could match any avulsed teeth you may have found.

Teeth that have been cleanly avulsed have a fair chance of being reattached if they are returned to their sockets within an hour or so, and the sooner the better. Try not to handle the tooth by its root—you will disturb the attachment fibers. Rinse the tooth in clean water and push it gently all the way back into its socket. You can splint the tooth to a healthy one adjacent to it by tying the two together with dental floss or fishing line. Any teeth that are very loose but still in the sockets may be splinted in this manner as well.

Fractured teeth that are still in place are often extremely sensitive on exposure to air if the nerve is still alive. The open site can be treated with a topical oral pain reliever like oil of cloves and covered temporarily with dental wax or Cavit, a temporary filling material that hardens on exposure to saliva. Cavit can be purchased without a prescription as part of an expensive commercially produced dental emergency kit. You could also ask your dentist for some at a cost of only a few dollars for a small jar.

The loss of a filling can be treated in the same way: Use wax or Cavit to protect the sensitive nerve tissue that is exposed when the filling falls out. If you're fresh out of Cavit, loose fillings or crowns can be temporarily glued back in place with toothpaste. The patient should eat only soft foods and drink only cool liquids.

Of course, any mouth held together with dental floss, wax, and toothpaste needs a dentist's attention as soon as possible. This need not be on an emergency basis unless pain cannot be controlled. With broken or avulsed teeth, infection is an important anticipated problem. Antibiotics, usually penicillin, are often given to prevent it.

ASSESSMENT OF DENTAL INFECTION

"Toothache" usually describes the pain experienced when an infection develops inside the tooth and at the base of the root. Bacteria enter through a break in the enamel caused by trauma or a cavity and form an abscess, with the typical swelling, pressure, and pain. Swelling of the gum on the affected side may be evident, as well as tenderness of one or more teeth when they are tapped with a finger or stick. The infection may remain localized or may spread into the adjacent bone or sinus. In either case, the patient will be extremely uncomfortable. Both dental infection and the pain it causes are difficult to manage in the field.

TREATMENT OF DENTAL INFECTION

The treatment of a dental infection includes drainage, antibiotics, and pain relief. Up until quite recently in dental history, drainage was invariably performed by pulling the tooth. The preferred method today is drilling and cleaning the inside of the tooth and installing a filling. Antibiotics are used to bring the infection under control, and pain relievers are usually necessary. What this means in the field is as simple as it is unfortunate: You need a dentist. Temporary pain relief may be obtained with oral topical pain relievers and aspirin or ibuprofen. If you carry antibiotics, a five- to seven-day course may reduce the severity of the infection pending evacuation to professional dental care.

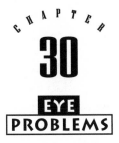

The common terms red eye, pink eye, or conjunctivitis refer to inflammation of the thin membranous lining of the eye and the inside of the eyelids (conjunctiva). There are a number of causes of conjunctival inflammation that can be treated in the field, but the inflammation can also represent one of the symptoms of a more serious condition such as glaucoma.

ASSESSMENT OF CONJUNCTIVITIS

All the various causes of conjunctivitis produce similar symptoms. The patient will complain of an itching or burning sensation, tearing, and photophobia (discomfort caused by bright light). The white of the eye will be covered with the enlarged blood vessels of the inflamed conjunctiva. In milder cases, the cornea will remain clear. The pupil will continue to react to light. Vision will be unaffected except for transient blurring caused by tears or yellow exudate. Normal eye movements might be uncomfortable but fully intact.

In more severe cases there may be clouding of the cornea, persistent visual disturbances, and severe headache. Causes of conjunctivitis include:

FOREIGN BODY.

Sand or other debris that gets onto the conjunctiva will cause immediate irritation, redness, and tearing. Onset is usually abrupt and the cause often obvious.

CORNEAL ABRASION.

The clear center structure of the eye can be scratched by a foreign body, branch, fingernail, or wind-blown ice crystals. It is exquisitely sensitive and will cause considerable pain and inflammation, making the patient feel like something is in the eye. Sometimes the abrasion will be visible by the light of a flashlight shining across the eye from the side.

SUNBURN.

Ultraviolet light can burn the conjunctiva and cornea as it does unprotected skin. The result is the same: pain, redness, and sometimes swelling. An exam will reveal that the inflammation is limited to the sun-exposed part of the eye, leaving the conjunctiva under the lids unaffected. In severe cases, the cornea may become pitted and cloudy in appearance.

INFECTION.

This is what most medical practitioners mean by the term "conjunctivitis." Bacteria invade the conjunctiva, causing the typical signs and symptoms of infection. The patient may notice yellow discharge that can glue the eyelids together during sleep. The eyelids themselves may appear slightly puffy and reddened.

CHEMICAL IRRITATION.

Soap, dirty contact lenses, stove fuel, all cause chemical conjunctivitis. In mild cases, the cornea remains clear. In severe cases it may be pitted or cloudy in appearance.

TREATMENT OF CONJUNCTIVITIS

Mild inflammation is usually easily treated in the field. If the cause is known, correct it, protect it, and allow it to heal.

FOREIGN BODY.

The easiest and least traumatic way to remove something from the eye is by irrigation with water. The simplest way to accomplish this is to have the patient immerse his face in clean water and blink his eyes. If there's no clean lake or stream handy, irrigate with your water bottle. Position him on his side with the affected eye up. Pour water gently on the lateral end of the eye and let it run across the eye toward the nose. Holding the lids open is not necessary if the patient can continue to blink during irrigation.

This technique will remove almost any object that lands in the eye. If the patient continues to have the sensation of something in there, you'll have to go looking for it. Gently pull the lids away from the eye one at a time while the patient looks in all directions. Look on the eye itself as well as on the conjunctival surface of the inside of the eye lids. A flashlight helps.

If you find something, use a wet cotton swab or corner of a gauze pad to lift it off the membrane. If the object is imbedded in the conjunctiva or cornea and resists your efforts to remove it, leave it alone. Imbedded foreign bodies require medical attention. Patch the eye, if it's safe to do so, and walk out. Beware of using a patch in situations where impaired vision could be dangerous.

CORNEAL ABRASION.

Abrasions will usually resolve on their own over the course of twenty-four hours. A patch may be used if it makes the patient more comfortable, but it is not necessary. Nonmedicated lubricating eye-drops will help relieve the pain of eye movement and can be used as often as desired.

SUNBURN.

Most inflammation from ultraviolet (UV) exposure is mild and self-limiting. However, if the damage is severe enough to cause cloudiness of the cornea or snow blindness, the eyes must be placed at rest and allowed to heal. Fortunately, UV rays do not penetrate deeply, so damage is usually superficial.

The treatment involves patching both eyes and keeping the patient rested and quiet. Pain medication may be necessary. Symptoms should resolve within twenty-four to forty-eight hours, after which the patient can safely be evacuated, if necessary.

INFECTION.

Most bacterial and viral conjunctivitis will resolve on its own, but this is difficult to predict. As with any infected tissue, allow the eyes to drain—do not use a patch. Some relief may be obtained through frequent rinsing and warm soaks. Treatment with antibiotics either orally or as eyedrops is the preferred treatment, especially if symptoms appear to become progressively worse rather than stabilizing or improving. Note also that a conjunctival infection can be quite contagious. Avoid sharing towels, goggles, or face masks.

CHEMICAL IRRITATION.

The treatment for chemical exposure is irrigation, and lots of it (thirty minutes minimum at a time). Expect mild redness following prolonged irrigation, but the condition should begin to resolve within several hours following treatment. If it gets worse, the chemical may still be present. Irrigation should be repeated and evacuation plans made.

Medicine

and

Medical Supplies

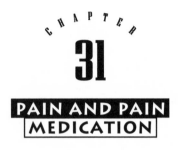

31

PAIN AND PAIN MEDICATION

Pain is essential to survival. It provides guidelines for the safe and efficient use of our bodies and functions as an early warning of serious trouble. It is the negative reinforcement that keeps us from doing bodily harm and serves to restrict mobility and prevent further damage after injury. It would be dangerous to eliminate pain completely.

The best treatment for pain is to treat its cause. Simple first-aid techniques will go a long way in pain relief. The body rewards good treatment by hurting less. The use of drugs to control pain should be viewed only as an adjunct to the definitive treatment of the basic problem.

Most analgesic (pain-relieving) medications can be divided into two general groups: narcotics and NSAIDS. Narcotics exert their analgesic effect on the central nervous system, relieving pain by suppressing the brain's ability to perceive it. Pain impulses are still being sent along the nerve pathways from the site of injury, but the intensity is dulled at the receiving end. Examples of narcotics include morphine, codeine, and meperidine (Demerol).

As a related effect, narcotics also depress mental function, respiration, and intestinal motility. When you're hurting, narcotics make you feel less pain, but they also make you stupid, clumsy, drowsy, and constipated. This may not be an issue in the comfort and safety of your own home, but it can be a real problem halfway across the Pacific or high in the mountains. Narcotics are certainly useful, but their risks often outweigh their benefits.

A better choice for most acute pain situations are the NSAIDS (nonsteroidal anti-inflammatory drugs), because they don't cause central nervous system depression. NSAIDS exert their pain-relieving effect at the site of injury by reducing the stimulation of pain receptors in peripheral nerves and by reducing inflammation and swelling. The brain is wide awake and able to perceive pain, but there are fewer pain impulses being sent. The granddaddy of all NSAIDS is aspirin, which is why NSAIDS are also referred to as aspirinlike drugs. Examples include ibuprofen (Advil, Nuprin), acetaminophen (Tylenol, Aspirin-Free Anacin), and naproxen sodium (Aleve).

Because NSAIDS are related to aspirin they are not given much credit as strong pain relievers. People just don't believe that something as easily available as aspirin could be very effective. But aspirin is an excellent pain reliever. So are ibuprofen and acetaminophen, which are often used in hospitals as the only post-surgery pain relievers necessary.

Injectable NSAIDS (for example, Toradol) offer pain relief equal to a hefty dose of morphine or meperidine (Demerol). But because they are not narcotic, they do not produce the typical narcotic buzz, drowsiness, or impaired mental function, and they do not depress respiration or blood pressure. For people skilled in performing injections, this kind of pain reliever is well worth considering as a substitute for narcotics. This is something you might want to discuss with your medical practitioner before any travel in a high-risk environment.

The primary undesirable side effect of NSAIDS is stomach irritation. The best way to avoid it is to always take NSAIDS with food or antacids. People with stomach problems should use these drugs with care, always taking the lowest effective dose. NSAIDS should be discontinued if persistent stomach pain develops.

The various NSAIDS available come in a broad spectrum of analgesic, anti-inflammatory, and antipyretic (antifever) properties. Ibuprofen does all three quite well and is a good choice for an expedition medical kit. It does a good job with minor to moderate pain at a dosage of 200–400 milligrams every eight hours but can be used at up to 800 milligrams every six hours for severe pain. Ibuprofen is often used to reduce swelling in sprains and tendinitis as well as to reduce fever in illness.

Acetaminophen is effective at relieving moderate pain and fever but is not useful for swelling and inflammation. It is still worth carrying because it tends to cause less stomach upset than other NSAIDS. Even people who can't take ibuprofen can usually tolerate acetaminophen.

Any pain medication should be used in the lowest effective dose for the shortest time necessary to minimize side effects. Always ask about allergies; people who are allergic to aspirin may react to any NSAID. Often, however, the patient will tell you that they can take Advil, Tylenol, or similar drugs without problems.

Finally, remember that medical information gets old quickly. New drugs, and new uses and contraindications for existing drugs, are being introduced all the time. As you stock your medical kit, supplement any published information by talking with a medical practitioner or pharmacist.

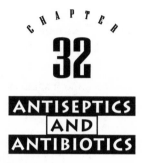

32

ANTISEPTICS AND ANTIBIOTICS

Antiseptics (also called disinfectants) are toxic chemicals that are designed to kill anything they come into contact with. Iodine and hydrogen peroxide are common examples. To control their effects, we adjust the concentration, site of application, and duration of contact. In low concentrations, antiseptics will do a nice job of killing bacteria, viruses, and amoebas without harming you.

In most cases the safest approach is to use low concentrations for long duration. This is the idea behind disinfecting drinking water with only a few drops of iodine per liter and leaving it to stand for thirty minutes. You can drink water purified in this manner for a long time with no ill effects.

For irrigating open wounds, I also prefer large quantities of a dilute solution of antiseptic, or just clean water. A concentrated solution would sterilize the wound faster and more completely, but it would kill lots of your body's cells in the process. The chances of wound infection would actually increase with all of those dead cells lying around.

"Full-strength" iodine solutions (Betadine, Povidone) are really only 2–10 percent strength, but this is enough to kill unprotected tissue. They should be used only to clean intact skin around a wound or before surgery and then should be washed off as soon as possible. Hydrogen peroxide is usually supplied as a 3 percent solution. It is less lethal than iodine but should not be used full strength in wounds either.

One of the best forms of antiseptic is iodine ointment (for example, Povidone iodine ointment). This is a low-concentration solution that can be left on a wound for long-term protection. The ointment is also water soluble, and a small dab will purify a liter of water for drinking or wound irrigation. It's a handy substance to have around.

The class of drugs known as antibiotics are a more sophisticated and selective way to kill bacteria. Their mechanism of action targets the specific life functions of a specific type of bacterial cell. Penicillin, for example, interferes with the ability of certain types of bacteria to construct new cell walls during reproduction. Although most antibiotics have side effects, killing large numbers of body cells is not one of them.

Individual antibiotics have a typical spectrum of activity; that is, they act against some bacteria but not others. Broad spectrum antibiotics act against a wide variety of bacteria and are more useful when you don't know exactly what you're dealing with. You can prepare to cover just about any type of infection on a remote expedition by carrying only two or three broad-spectrum antibiotics in your kit. Because bacteria rapidly develop resistance to antibiotics, a particular drug's effectiveness will change monthly, and new drugs are constantly being introduced. Ask an experienced medical practitioner for current recommendations.

One of the most useful ways to use antibiotics is in the form of antibiotic ointment (for example, Bacitracin), which is available without prescription. It is used to treat or prevent superficial skin infections without damaging healing skin cells. Unlike iodine ointment, it cannot purify water.

Unfortunately, although antibiotics are useful against cellular organisms like bacteria and amoebas, they don't do a thing to your garden variety virus. You can take penicillin until you're blue in the face and it won't help you get rid of a cold. There are currently very few drugs that are effective against viruses, and those that are available tend to be extremely expensive.

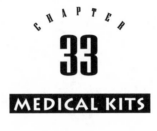

33

MEDICAL KITS

The marketing departments of most outdoor equipment suppliers count on the medical naïveté of the general public and on our tendency to try to solve most problems with money. Dozens of types of medical kits are offered, most at prices vastly inflated over the value of their contents. You may be able to do a lot better on your own.

By now, you know that the most important element of any first-aid kit is the knowledge and experience you carry in your head. The equipment and supplies you need can be relatively simple and inexpensive. How much first-aid equipment you carry is a function of how you carry it, how many people you're responsible for, where you're going, and what you know.

There is no point in carrying anything you don't know how to use. If you're carrying it on your back, there is no reason to carry anything that can be improvised from something else. As a result, a first-aid kit for backpacking can be about the size of this book. Larger groups, or people traveling by vehicle, boat, or horse have the luxury of carrying more complete supplies.

On most trips it makes sense to arrange your kit in modules. Put the materials used for minor maintenance and repair, like Band-

Aids and moleskin, in a separate container. This module will have as much to do with preventing medical problems as treating them, and should be easily accessible. It may work best for each person in a group to have his or her own. Because this part of the kit will get a lot of use and be the most exposed to damage from snow and rain, it should contain few supplies. It can be replenished from the main expedition kit as needed.

Medications, like antibiotics and pain relievers, should be in another module, preferably in a crushproof, waterproof, plastic box. It should contain instructions and precautions for the use of the drugs carried, as well as a small notebook for recording times and dosages. Any prescription medications should be accompanied by documentation from the prescribing practitioner, especially if you will be crossing international borders. In large groups it should be carried by the trip leader or medical officer.

The largest module is the main expedition kit. Because it serves mostly as a supply dump for the smaller modules, its size depends on the length of the trip. It should also include infrequently used and specialized first-aid supplies and equipment. The type of container you put it in will be determined by how you travel. The ubiquitous five-gallon joint-compound bucket has performed beautifully as a waterproof container on Outward Bound pulling boats. A compressible dry bag is good for pack or hiking trips. In wet conditions, it's a good idea to further protect supplies inside the main kit by dividing them into several plastic bags.

Your local pharmacist can be a great resource in acquiring supplies. She can also help you put medications into vials much smaller than the original packaging. A pharmacist should also be willing to point out generic medications that are equivalents to the expensive brand-name stuff. Go in with your whole supply list, explain what you're doing, and ask for a bulk discount.

The following list is a recommended basic kit. You will need to modify it to suit the conditions you expect and your level of training, but resist the temptation to load up on a lot of unnecessary gear. Your expedition medical kit is an integral part of your whole gear inventory and trip plan, not a stand-alone item. You don't need to weigh your kit down with hot packs, cold packs, triangular bandages, air splints, flashlights, and signal mirrors, the stuff that makes the commercial kits so big and expensive. Most of the splints and slings can be improvised, and you are already carrying the "survival gear."

EXPEDITION MEDICAL KIT

MODULE ONE.

Knowledge and experience. Invest in at least a weekend of training in backcountry or marine medicine.

MODULE TWO.

Reference. Carry written material like this book and others, that you like and understand. You can tear out and carry only the important pages.

MODULE THREE.

Minor maintenance and repair kit:

Sterile scalpel blade

2 4x4-inch sterile gauze dressings

2 2x2-inch sterile gauze dressings

1 2x2-inch gel dressing or moleskin for blisters

6 Band-Aids (The flexible type is best.)

1 roll 1-inch flexible adhesive tape (Conforms to and moves with the body.)

1 small bottle or ampule of tincture of benzoin (Makes the skin sticky to hold tape in wet or cold weather.)

1 small tube Povidone iodine ointment (Antiseptic for abrasions, burns, and blisters. A small dab dissolved in a quart of water purifies it for drinking or wound irrigation.)

1 small bottle liquid soap

1 pair splinter forceps (Small tweezers.)

1-gallon plastic bag (Holds water for irrigating wounds; poke a small hole in the bottom to make it squirt.)

2-inch elastic bandage (Used to hold dressings in place over wounds, or as compression bandage.)

At least 4 pair latex gloves

Sunblock

Insect repellent

MODULE FOUR.

Medications:

Nonprescription

Small bottle of acetaminophen (Tylenol)

Small bottle of ibuprofen (Advil)

Stool softener, (e.g., Colase)

Package of Pepto-Bismol tablets

Package of antacid tablets

Cough and cold preparations as desired

Diphenhydramine capsules (Benadryl)

Dramamine or other medication for motion sickness

Vitamin C

Prescription (Discuss with your medical practitioner.)

Antibiotic tablets

Antibiotic eye ointment or drops

Epinephrine kit for severe allergy (Anakit, Epipen)

Medication for severe pain

Medication for vomiting and diarrhea

Steroid cream

Diamox (If going to altitude.)

Malaria prophylaxis if needed

MODULE FIVE.

Main expedition kit:

Resupply materials for Module Three kits (Adjust quantities to size of group.)

SAM Splint (Flexible aluminum covered with foam, can be cut and bent for a variety of uses. The only splint worth carrying on your back.)

4 diaper pins

Elastic bandage, 4-inch and 6-inch (Good for wound care and compression as well as improvised splinting.)

Large dressings for big wounds (Sanitary napkins work well.)

Xeroform gauze dressings (A foil-wrapped dressing impregnated with antiseptic that is especially useful in the long-term care of open wounds.)

Dental kit (Oil of cloves, Cavit from your dentist, dental wax, toothpaste, dental floss.)

100 feet of 6-millimeter low-stretch rope (If not carried elsewhere.)

Roll of 15 yards of duct tape (For litters and splints, also fixes tents, boots, and boats.)

A handful of big plastic cable ties (For improvised litters and general repair.)

1 pair trauma scissors (Cuts almost anything, including SAM Splint.)

1 fine hemostat (Good for picking rocks and dirt from wounds or extracting hooks from humans or fish.)

Low-reading clinical thermometer

Burn sheet (100 percent cotton T-shirt fresh from the dryer, kept in a plastic bag.)

Notebook and pencil

Butane lighter (Warms duct tape to make it stick well in cold weather.)

DAY USE PERSONAL FIRST-AID KIT (FITS IN A HUNTING COAT POCKET)

1 roll 1-inch adhesive tape

2 4x4-inch gauze pads

1 large dressing (Sanitary napkin works well.)

1 3-inch elastic bandage

5 Band-Aids

1 3x3-inch blister pad such as Spenco Adhesive Knit or mole-skin

1 pair latex examination gloves

2 diaper pins

1 pair splinter forceps

1 emergency flashlight if not carried elsewhere

1 lighter, or waterproof matches

1 knife if not carried elsewhere

1 small container of liquid soap

1 tube of Povidone iodine ointment

1 container of total sunblock

1 5-yard role of duct tape

4 200-milligram ibuprofen tablets

SECTION VIII

Wilderness

Travel

34

PREPARATION FOR WILDERNESS EMERGENCIES

The traditional view holds that the best preparation for medical emergencies is not to have them in the first place. I agree. There are plenty of how-to books on camping, sailing, canoeing, ice climbing, and so forth to help you do it right. Read them.

But because medical emergencies are what *this* book is about, I'll take the statement a step farther: The best time to have a medical emergency is when you're ready for it. Being ready means having the right attitude, knowledge, equipment, and margin of safety for the expedition or voyage you're planning.

Attitude, in my view, is the way one relates with the forces of the natural world. It is so much more peaceful to flow with natural trends than to push against them. However, it is not always possible to go downriver, downhill, downwind, or with the tide. We tend to have schedules, destinations, and personal goals that put us in opposition to nature.

Of course, challenging the elements can be great fun and an exhilarating experience. As long as you continue to feel that way, you'll be OK. However, one must beware of developing an adverse relationship with nature. This is a forewarning of serious trouble.

When it starts raining on *you,* or the wind shifts just to make *you* angry, or the snow starts just because *it* knows *you're* almost at the summit, your attitude has become dangerous. In an emergency situation, a bad attitude contributes to irrational behavior, poor judgment, despair—and big trouble. When you feel the attitude, it's time to change your plans and reestablish harmony with your surroundings.

Knowing how to handle medical emergencies is a product of information and experience. Only by combining the two can you gain real competence in the art of wilderness medicine. The information you need is available in this book and in others like it. The experience is more difficult to come by. A reasonable substitute, at least as a beginning, can be found in the form of a quality hands-on first-aid course that focuses on wilderness situations.

Knowing what to expect of the environment you are entering is also important. You need to research expected weather and terrain conditions and be aware of the possible extreme situations you might confront. You should identify possible evacuation routes in case of trouble and establish some means of communication. You will want to know where shelters, ranger stations, roads, water, and so forth are located.

Equipment for wilderness emergency care is surprisingly simple. The real first-aid kit is your knowledge and experience. The bandages, ointments, moleskin, and other items in your pack are just tools for minor maintenance and repair.

The margin of safety in wilderness travel is the most important factor of all. An accident or illness that befalls a group that is dry, warm, and well fed is a problem but usually not a crisis. But if the group is wet, chilled, and low on supplies, the situation could be entirely different. Even a minor injury at that point can easily be fatal.

When you're in the mountains, out to sea, or on the river, you should frequently ask yourself, "What would I do if something went wrong?" It sounds a little paranoid, but this is a great exercise for the traveler new to the backcountry. If your answers are not coming up clear and reasonable, you are beyond your margin of safety. As you gain experience, you will become acutely aware of your own margin of safety. You feel comfortable within it and uneasy outside it. Pushing your own limits then becomes a matter of choice rather than accident.

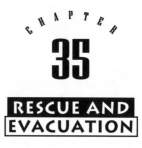

CHAPTER
35
RESCUE AND EVACUATION

As I review my writing, I realize how many times treatment plans call for "evacuation to medical care," as if it were as easy as catching a bus. In reality, it is everything but easy, especially when the injured person is no longer able to walk. A wilderness rescue can be a most dangerous and difficult operation.

Outside of state and national parks and a few municipalities, there is little in the way of organized professional response to back-country emergencies. Depending on where you are located, the responsibility for wilderness rescue is assumed by a variety of officials, which might include the Warden Service, Coast Guard, or local fire departments, police, or ambulance crews. The official response usually relies heavily on volunteer rescue teams, the National Guard, ski patrols, and other organizations and individuals to do the actual work.

In some cases a rescue will be a well-coordinated effort by competent officials and well-trained volunteers. In others the effort can be disorganized, inefficient, and downright dangerous. Either situation can occur depending on where you are, the situation you're in, and even the day of the week.

In spite of this inconsistency, it is not a situation that merits much complaint. As backcountry travelers and offshore sailors, we represent a minuscule portion of the general population. It is difficult to justify maintaining a sophisticated and expensive wilderness rescue system for so few people. This means that to enter the wilderness is to accept a much greater degree of personal responsibility. We must be able to get ourselves out of trouble whenever possible. Lacking that, we must be able to be of the greatest possible assistance to those who are coming to help us.

When you have stabilized a medical problem as best you can and have decided that outside help will be required, your communication skills become critical. Presenting a clear picture of the situation will allow rescuers to best apply their own local knowledge, experience, and resources to helping *you* solve *your* problem. This is where your SOAP note really becomes valuable. Not only has it helped you organize your thoughts, but it can now provide the basis for organizing an evacuation. This is true whether you communicate by radio, telephone, carrier pigeon, or by sending a runner with a note.

Your SOAP note should include information about the scene. Describe the general condition of the group, weather and terrain conditions, and the status of food supplies and shelter. Try to stick to facts as much as possible. Avoid value judgments like: "Oh my God, it's really bad, come quick!" These provide no useful information and only distract people from a good planning process.

Recognize that any good rescue team is trained to perform its own survey of the scene and the patient's condition. The team's assessment may differ from yours. Don't argue. Work with the team, pointing out elements of your assessment that will help form a reasonable plan. Remember: When you've asked for rescue, the rescuers are in charge in all but the most unusual cases.

Responding to a medical emergency can be done by bringing the medical resources to the patient or the patient to the medicine. Usually it is a combination of the two. For example, rescue teams may bring intravenous fluids and oxygen to assist in stabilizing a patient during the carry-out. For the most part, though, the patient needs to return to civilization for definitive care.

The urgency with which this happens is a function of the patient's condition and the resources and skills available. It also hinges on your ability to distinguish real emergencies from logistical dilemmas. Very few backcountry situations really justify an all-out rapid evacuation. Only those injuries that involve a major problem with a major body system deserve a major evacuation. Anything else can be more controlled, less desperate, and a lot less trouble.

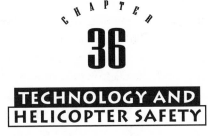

36

TECHNOLOGY AND HELICOPTER SAFETY

The recent proliferation of cell phone and radio technology and the full activation of the Global Positioning System (GPS) has created a revolution in the business of backcountry rescue. If you know how to use the equipment, it is possible to know exactly where you've been, where you are, and where you're going and to be able to tell the whole world about it. The downside of this is that a lot of backcountry users, and some rescue teams, are substituting technology for skill and common sense. Reinforced by the entertainment media, there is a popular perception that all you need to do to get out of trouble is to flip open your cell phone and whistle up a helicopter.

Unfortunately, for all their glamour, helicopters are the most expensive and dangerous rescue technology we have. Aeromedical helicopters are some of the most accident-prone ships in the air, and wilderness search and rescue is one of the most dangerous things a pilot can do. The risk-to-benefit ratio seldom favors their use, and the backcountry traveler or ocean voyager should never plan on them as a first line of salvation.

In spite of its obvious drawbacks, helicopter use in medical evacuation and search and rescue is expanding. It is still sometimes the best tool available, and you should know something about it. Though helicopter safety is a subject large enough to have its own textbooks, there are a few basic precautions worthy of mention here.

Although helicopters are capable of dropping straight down from a hovering position, this is a very difficult maneuver. The pilot will prefer to approach a landing zone (or helispot) from downwind with some forward speed. The approach must be free of electrical wires, tall trees, and other obstacles. Because the pilot will prefer to lift forward into the wind, the take-off direction should also be clear. The best information you can give a pilot from the ground is the location of obstacles and the direction of the wind. If you don't have voice communication, don't choose a landing zone with obstacles that might be difficult for the pilot to see.

Streamers made from lightweight fabric tied to trees can be used to indicate wind direction. A trained rescue team will employ a "parking tender" who is positioned to indicate wind direction and give hand signals to help the pilot on approach. If you're not comfortable with the hand signals yourself, don't confuse the pilot by inventing your own. Keep your arms down unless you see a problem.

If you *do* see a problem, the "wave off" is the universal signal for "get out of here." The hands are repeatedly crossed above your head, just as you would do instinctively to attract attention or summon help. To the pilot this means "go away" or "danger." You can see the potential for confusion here: Don't wave at a helicopter unless you want it to leave.

On its landing approach a helicopter will kick up a hurricane of dust or snow. Secure everything, stay well clear, and resist the temptation to watch it land unless you are wearing goggles and can keep your mouth shut. The pilot may shut down the engine or keep the rotors turning while the helicopter is on the ground depending on the situation. Needless to say, a running helicopter represents a significant hazard.

Most helicopters have a large horizontal lift rotor overhead that is generally high enough to walk under and a small vertical tail rotor that is generally low enough to cut you into little pieces. Always approach these craft forward of amidships, and only after getting an

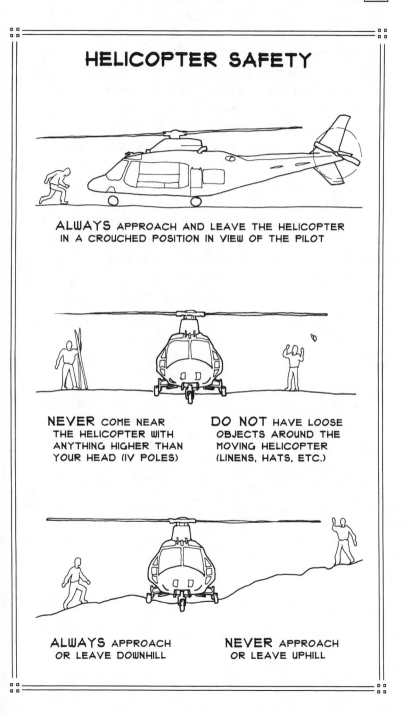

HELICOPTER SAFETY

ALWAYS APPROACH AND LEAVE THE HELICOPTER
IN A CROUCHED POSITION IN VIEW OF THE PILOT

NEVER COME NEAR
THE HELICOPTER WITH
ANYTHING HIGHER THAN
YOUR HEAD (IV POLES)

DO NOT HAVE LOOSE
OBJECTS AROUND THE
MOVING HELICOPTER
(LINENS, HATS, ETC.)

ALWAYS APPROACH
OR LEAVE DOWNHILL

NEVER APPROACH
OR LEAVE UPHILL

OK from the pilot. Stoop low to maximize the distance between your head and the rotor blades, and carry any equipment or packs low and in front of you. If the helicopter is on a slope, approach only from the downhill side and in full view of the pilot. If in doubt, the safest way to approach a running helicopter is at the side of a crew member or trained rescuer.

If you are involved in a hoist operation, remember not to be the first ground contact with the hoist cable. The friction of air against the rotor blades generates a significant electrostatic charge that will be discharged through the first thing the cable touches. Let it touch the ground, sea, or steel deck before you handle it. Also, because the aircraft could rise suddenly with wind gusts, never secure the cable to anything you do not intend to hoist immediately.

Again, helicopter safety is a broad topic. If you anticipate working around these machines, read the appropriate references and get the appropriate training.

APPENDIX I

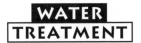

The word "disinfect" means to kill or remove living organisms like bacteria, protozoans, algae, and viruses. "To purify" implies removing all foreign material, including chemicals and minerals, as well as life, a much more difficult process. In the wilderness setting, where surface water is not subject to industrial contamination, our goal is usually just to eliminate disease-causing microorganisms.

1. Boil: Just bringing water to a boil disinfects it enough for drinking.

2. Chemicals: Double the standing time if the water is cold. Double the dose if the water is cloudy.

   a. Iodine Tincture (2%): Use two to five drops of tincture per quart of water and let it stand for thirty minutes.

   b. Iodine Tablets: Use one tablet per quart of water and let it stand for thirty minutes.

   c. Chlorine: Use two drops of pure laundry bleach per quart of water and let it stand for thirty minutes.

3. Filters: To prevent clogging, prefilter the water through a cloth to remove large sediment. Note: The typical .2-micron

filter will trap larger organisms like bacteria and giardia, but does not remove viruses (for instance, hepatitis). If the filter you are using does not include a virucidal agent like an iodine cartridge, treat any water subject to fecal contamination with iodine or chlorine. Activated charcoal filters are capable of removing some chemical pollutants and sediment not affected by boiling. They will also remove the taste of chlorine or iodine after disinfection.

APPENDIX II

COMMON ABBREVIATIONS

ALS   Advanced Life Support
AVPU
            Awake
            Verbal stimulus response
            Painful stimulus response
            Unresponsive
BLS   Basic Life Support
CNS   Central nervous system
CPR   Cardiopulmonary resuscitation
CSM   Circulation, sensation, movement
CVA   Cerebrovascular accident
EMS   Emergency Medical Services
HACE   High altitude cerebral edema
HAPE   High altitude pulmonary edema
Hx   History
ICP   Intracranial pressure
IV   Intravenous
MAST   Military Anti-Shock Trousers
MI   Myocardial infarction (heart attack)

MOI	Mechanism of injury
O$_2$	Oxygen
PAS	Patient Assessment System
PFA	Pain-free activity
RF	Red flag
RICE	
	Rest
	Ice
	Compression
	Elevation
Rx	Treatment
SAMPLE	
	Symptoms
	Allergies
	Medication
	Past history of medical problems
	Last food and fluids
	Events leading to injury
SOAP	
	Subjective: information gained by questioning
	Objective: information gathered during examination of the patient
	Assessment: list of problems discovered
	Plan: what is to be done about each problem
SOB	Shortness of breath
S/SX	Signs/symptoms
TIP	Traction into position
VS	Vital signs (with time recorded):
	BP blood pressure
	R respiratory rate
	T core temperature
	C level of consciousness (mental status if awake)
	S skin
	P pulse

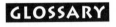

GLOSSARY

Abrasion: A superficial wound that damages only the outermost layers of skin or cornea.

Abscess: An infection that has been isolated from the rest of the body by inflammation.

Ace Bandage: The brand name of an elastic bandage that is used to apply compression to an injured extremity.

Acute Stress Reaction (ASR): Autonomic-nervous-system-controlled response to stress that can cause severe but temporary and reversible changes in vital signs.

Airway: The passage for air movement from the nose and mouth through the throat to the lungs.

Altitude sickness: Also known as acute mountain sickness. Primarily the symptoms associated with the effects of oxygen deprivation on the brain occurring at high altitudes. Can be mild, moderate, or severe.

Alveoli: Membranous air sacs in the lungs where gas is exchanged with the blood.

Anaphylaxis: Systemic allergic reaction involving generalized edema of all body surfaces and vascular shock.

Anticipated problems (A'): Problems that may develop over time as a result of injury, illness, or the environment.

Aspiration: Inhaling foreign liquid or other material into the lungs.

Basic Life Support (BLS): The generic process of supporting the functions of the circulatory, respiratory, and nervous systems using artificial ventilation, chest compressions, bleeding control, and spinal immobilization.

Capillaries: The smallest blood vessels in body tissues where gases and nutrients are exchanged between tissue cells and the circulating blood.

Cardiac arrest: Loss of effective heart activity.

Cardiogenic shock: Shock due to inadequate pumping action of the heart.

Cardiopulmonary Resuscitation (CPR): A technique for artificially circulating oxygenated blood in the absence of effective heart activity. Includes artificial respiration and chest compressions.

Carotid pulse: The pulse felt on the side of the neck at the site of the carotid artery.

Cartilage: Connective tissue on the ends of bones at joints. It provides a smooth gliding surface.

Cavit: The brand name of a temporary dental filling material that hardens on exposure to saliva.

Central nervous system: The brain and spinal cord.

Cervical spine: The section of the spine in the neck between the base of the skull and the top of the thorax.

Cold challenge: The combined cooling influence of wind, humidity, and ambient temperature.

Cold response: The normal body response to the cold challenge, including the shell/core effect and shivering.

Compartment syndrome: Swelling within a confined body compartment, such as the connective tissue compartments in the leg or arm, that develops enough pressure to cause ischemia and may result in death of tissue.

Compensation: Involuntary changes in body functions designed to maintain perfusion of vital body tissues in the presence of injury or illness.

Conjunctiva: The membrane covering the white of the eye and the inner surfaces of the eyelids.

Conjunctivitis: Inflammation of the conjunctiva due to irritation, infection, or injury. Also known as red eye.

Cornea: The clear part of the eye over the iris and pupil.

Cornice: An overhanging drift of snow formed as wind blows over a ridge or mountaintop.

Crepitus: The grating or crunching of broken bones or cartilage felt with movement.

Dental abscess: Infection at the base of a tooth.

Diagnosis: The specific identification of an illness or injury by name.

Diaphragm: The muscle at the lower end of the chest cavity, which, when contracting, creates a vacuum that draws air into the lungs. The diaphragm works with muscles of the chest wall, shoulders, and neck to perform ventilation.

Disability: In the Initial Assessment, loss or potential loss of central nervous system function due to brain or spinal cord injury.

Discharge: Fluid escaping from the site of infection or inflammation.

Dislocation: Disruption of normal joint anatomy.

Distal: An anatomical direction—away from the body center.

Edema: Swelling due to the leakage of serum from capillaries.

Epinephrine: The synthetic form of the hormone adrenaline. A vaso-constricting drug.

Evacuation: Removing a patient from the scene of injury or illness, usually en route to medical care.

Extension: Movement of a joint that takes the extremity away from the body. The opposite of flexion.

Exudate: Discharge.

Femoral artery: A large artery that travels along the femur in the thigh.

Femur: The long bone of the thigh.

Flail chest: The loss of rigidity of the chest wall due to injury involving multiple fractured ribs.

Flexion: Movement of a joint that brings the extremity closer to the body. The opposite of extension.

Focused History and Physical Exam: The stage in the Patient Assessment System that includes examining the whole body, taking the SAMPLE History, and recording the vital signs.

Fracture: Broken bone or cartilage.

Frostbite: Frozen tissue.

Frostnip: Loss of circulation due to the vasoconstriction of blood vessels in the skin during the early stages of tissue freezing.

Glaucoma: Disease or condition causing increased pressure within the globe of the eye.

Head injury: Injury to the brain.

Heart attack: An episode of heart muscle ischemia caused by a blood clot or spasm of the coronary arteries.

Heat challenge: Combined effects of ambient temperature and metabolic activity, which contribute to body heating.

Heat exhaustion: Compensated volume shock caused by fluid loss due to sweating.

Heat response: The normal body response to the heat challenge, including sweating and vasodilation of the shell.

Heat stroke: Severe elevation of body temperature (over 105 degrees Fahrenheit).

Hemothorax: Free blood in the chest cavity, usually from injury.

Hyperextension: To extend a joint beyond its normal range of motion.

Hyperventilation syndrome: The symptoms caused by reduced carbon dioxide in the blood due to excessive ventilation, usually associated with Acute Stress Reaction.

Hyperthermia: An abnormal increase in body core temperature. Above 105 degrees Fahrenheit may be considered life threatening.

Hypothermia: Below normal body-core temperature (96 degrees Fahrenheit). Can be mild (less than 96 degrees) or severe (less than 90 degrees).

Infection: Colonization of body tissues by bacteria, viruses, or other microorganisms.

Inflammatory process: A generic body response to illness or injury resulting in redness, swelling, warmth, and tenderness.

Initial Assessment: The first examination of an injured patient that includes assessment of airway, breathing, circulation, and disability.

Intoxicated: Altered level of consciousness or mental status due to the influence of chemicals such drugs, alcohol, and inhaled gases.

Intracranial: Inside the skull (cranium).

Ischemia: Lack of local perfusion to body tissues.

IV fluids: Fluids infused directly into the circulatory system through a hypodermic needle inserted into a vein. Usually used to temporarily increase the volume of circulating blood.

Level of consciousness: Describes the level of brain function in terms of responsiveness to specific stimuli. Measured by the AVPU scale: A, awake; V, responds to verbal stimuli; P, responds to painful stimuli; U, unresponsive to any stimuli.

Ligaments: Tough connective tissue joining bone to bone across joints.

Local effects: Effects that are restricted to the immediate area of injury or infection.

Lower airway: The trachea, bronchi, and alveoli.

Long bones: Bones that have a long structural axis, for instance, leg and arm bones, as opposed to flat bones like the ribs and shoulder blades.

Lumbar spine: The lower section of the spine, between the thorax and the pelvis.

Mechanism of injury: The cause of injury, or a description of the forces involved.

Mental status: Describes the level of brain function in an alert patient (A on the AVPU scale) in terms of memory, level of anxiety, and behavior.

Midrange position: A position in a joint's range of motion between full extension and full flexion.

Monitor: Regularly repeated patient assessment for the purpose of revising assessments and plans as the situation changes.

Near drowning: At least temporary survival of water inhalation. Usually associated with the protective effects of hypothermia in cold water.

Neutral position: The muscle position approximately halfway between flexion and extension.

Open fracture: A fracture with an associated break in the skin.

Oxygenation: Saturation of blood with oxygen. Oxygenation of the blood takes place in the lungs.

Patella: The kneecap.

Patient Assessment System: A system of surveys including Scene Size-up, Initial Assessment, and Focused History and Physical Exam designed to gather information about injured or ill patients and the environment in which they are found.

Penicillin: An antibiotic drug.

Perfusion: The passage of blood through capillary beds in body tissues.

Photophobia: Eye pain or headache caused by bright lights.

Pneumonia: Infection of lung tissue.

Pneumothorax: Free air in the chest cavity, usually from a punctured lung or chest wall.

Pulmonary edema: Swelling of lung tissue resulting in the collection of fluid in the alveoli.

Reduction: Restoring a dislocated joint to its normal position. Also, restoring a displaced fracture to normal anatomic position.

Scene Size-up: The stage of the Patient Assessment System during which one looks for dangers to the rescuer and patient, the number of people injured, and the mechanism of injury.

Seizures: Uncoordinated electrical activity in the brain.

Serum: The liquid portion of the blood, as distinguished from blood cells and platelets.

Sexually transmitted disease (STD): An infection transmitted from person to person by sexual activity.

Shell/core effect: A compensatory mechanism seen in shock and cold response that reduces blood flow to the body shell in order to preserve perfusion and warmth in the vital organs of the core.

Shock: Inadequate perfusion pressure due to a circulatory system problem such as blood loss, dehydration, or an injured heart.

Signs: A response elicited by examination. For example, pain or tenderness when the examiner touches an injured area.

Sinus: Hollow spaces in the bones of the skull.

Sinusitis: Inflammation of the membranous lining of the sinuses, usually due to infection.

Spasm: Involuntary contraction of muscle.

Spinal cord: The cordlike extension of the central nervous system encased within the bones of the spinal column and running from the base of the brain to the midlumbar spine.

Spine: The column of bony vertebrae extending from the base of the skull to the pelvis.

Stethoscope: An instrument used to transmit body sounds directly to the ears of the examiner through rubber tubes.

Survey: A systematic physical examination.

Swelling: Abnormal fluid accumulation in body tissues due to injury or illness.

Symptoms: A condition described by the patient: for example, pain on swallowing.

Systemic: Involving the entire body.

Tetanus: A disease caused by the toxins released by *Clostridium tetani* bacterium that may infect wounds (lockjaw).

Thorax: The region of the body between the base of the neck and the top of the abdomen; the chest.

Tourniquet: A constricting band used to prevent or restrict the flow of blood to an extremity.

Toxin load: The combined systemic effect of numerous small toxic exposures, for instance, a large number of insect bites or jellyfish stings.

Toxins: Chemicals that have a damaging effect on body tissues or the function of the nervous system.

Traction: Tension applied along the long axis of an extremity.

Traction splint: A splinting device designed to maintain traction on an extremity; used for femur fractures.

Trauma: Injury

Trench Foot: Inflammation due to the tissue damage that results from the prolonged constriction of blood vessels in tissues exposed to above-freezing cold and wet conditions for a long period of time.

Upper airway: The mouth, nose, and throat.

Vapor barrier: A vaporproof wrap or covering that prevents evaporative cooling.

Vascular bundle: A nerve, artery, and vein following the same pathway.

Vascular shock: Shock due to dilation of blood vessels.

Ventilation: The movement of air in and out of the lungs.

Vertebrae: The bones of the spine.

Vital signs: Measurements of body function including blood pressure, pulse, respiration, level of consciousness, skin color, and body-core temperature.

FURTHER READING

Auerbach, Paul S., M.D. *Medicine for the Outdoors*. Little, Brown, and Company, 1991.

Dickson, Murry. *Where There Is No Dentist*. The Hesperian Foundation, 1993.

Feinstein, Alice, ed. *Symptoms, Their Causes and Cures*. Rodale Press, Inc., 1994.

Forgey, William, M.D., ed. *Wilderness Medical Society Practice Guidelines for Wilderness Emergency Care*. ICS Books, 1995.

Goth, Peter, M.D. *Spine Injury; Clinical Criteria for Assessment and Management*. Medical Care Development, Inc., 1995.

The Hurricane Island Outward Bound School. *The Instructor's Field Manual*. 1993.

Krakauer, Jon. *Into the Wild*. Villard, 1996.

Morrissey, James. *The Wilderness Medical Associates Field Guide*. Wilderness Medical Associates, Inc., 1997.

Schimelpfenig, Tod, and Linda Lindsey. *NOLS Wilderness First Aid*. Stackpole Books, 1991.

Stewart, Charles E., M.D. *Environmental Emergencies*. Williams and Wilkins, 1990.

Weiss, Hal. *Secrets of Warmth*. Cloudcap, 1992.

Werner, David. *Where There Is No Doctor*. The Hesperian Foundation, 1992.

ACKNOWLEDGMENTS

This book is the result of a basic idea that has enjoyed years of refinement, elaboration, and critique by hundreds of generous and thoughtful people. My appreciation is extended to all of those individuals and organizations who have contributed their expertise and knowledge over the years. In particular, I would like to thank my fellow Outward Bound instructors and support staff for all of their comments, suggestions, and advice. I would also like to acknowledge the exceptional contributions made by the Sunday River and Sugarloaf Mountain Ski Patrols to the depth of knowledge and field experience presented here.

Most notable is Dr. Peter Goth, my mentor and coauthor for the first edition, and chief advisor, critic, and guardian of common sense for this one. I am deeply indebted to him for his experience, philosophy, and teaching principles and publications, which serve as the foundation for much of this book. I would also like to extend my heartfelt thanks to David Johnson, Jim Morrissey, Dennis Karrigan, Ben Woodard, Gretchen and Phil Gormley, and the rest of the staff of Wilderness Medical Associates for generously sharing their experience, comments, encouragement, and teaching materials. Laura Wininger, my wife, has earned my eternal gratitude and admiration for her efforts to illustrate this book so well, and for her patience and good humor with a process that tied up the computer for months, and scattered papers around the house like autumn leaves.

Jeffrey Isaac, P.A.-C.

INDEX

pneumonia, 50, 165, 166
pneumothorax, 52
poisons. *See* toxins
"positive mechanism" (patient
        assessment), 33–34
positive pressure ventilation (PPV),
        28, 30, 31, 53, 170
psychogenic shock, 9, 40
"puddle vision," 13
pulmonary edema, 7, 50–51,
        165–66, 191
pulse rate, 4, 17, 30–31, 38, 77
puncture wounds, 108, 110, 111
pus, 109–10, 115

quadriplegia, 92

radial (wrist) artery, 17
ragged wounds, 110
rectal temperature, 18, 150
repetitive motion injuries, 102
rescue operations, xv–xvi, 8, 172,
        228–30. *See also* emergencies;
        evacuations
    helicopters in, 231–32, 233, 234
rescuers, safety of, 12–13
respiratory arrest, 53, 92, 168–69,
        170
respiratory burns, 119
respiratory distress, 47, 56, 118, 119,
        126
respiratory failure, 159, 160, 173
respiratory infection, 202–3
respiratory rate, 4, 17–18, 38
respiratory system, 2, 3, 10, 45–56,
        46, 117, 150
rib fractures, 52–53
ribs, 71
RICE (rest, ice, elevation, compres-
        sion), 100, 101
risk/benefit ratio, 8, 8

safety, xii–xiii, 12–13

safety pins, 81
salt replacement, 142
SAMPLE list (patient history), 19,
        20
SAM Splint, 82, 97, 222
scene size-up, 12–13, 169
second-degree burns, 118
seizures, 63–64
sensation, loss of, 77, 156
separations, dislocations and, 86
septic shock, 116
severe blood loss, 32, 108
severe hypothermia, 150–52
severe sprains, 75
sexually transmitted disease, 198
shallow wounds, 108, 121
shell/core effect, 4, 4, 38, 41, 141,
        145, 146, 148, 154, 156, 165
shock, 31, 33, 37–40, 126, 143, 145,
        170, 181
shoulder dislocations, 84–89, 85,
        86, 88
simple fractures, 74
sinusitis, 193–94
skin, 4, 6
skin and soft tissue injuries, 106–23,
        127
skin color and warmth, 4, 18
snakebites, 129–31
SOAP (Subjective, Objective,
        Assessment, Plan), 20–23,
        229
soft tissue, 107, 111
solid organs, 179–81
speech, loss of, 63
spinal cord, 10, 57, 72, 73
    injury to, 29, 30, 32, 33–34, 38,
        65, 92–97, 96
spleen, 180
splints, 66, 70, 81–82, 83, 84,
        91–92, 97, 98, 103, 112, 113,
        220
sprains, 73

ABOUT THE AUTHOR

Jeff Isaac is a licensed physician assistant with a particular interest in backcountry and marine medicine. His professional experience includes service as an ambulance and rescue crewman, professional ski patroller, and twelve years as the director and medical staff member of a busy ski area trauma clinic. His "off season" is spent moonlighting in hospital emergency departments, and as a senior instructor and vessel master with the Hurricane Island Outward Bound School. He is a licensed captain, and an experienced blue water sailor, having logged thousands of miles aboard his 31-foot sloop, *October*, as well as sail training and oceanographic research vessels.

While teaching on Hurricane Island in 1982, Jeff met with Dr. Peter Goth around the challenge of designing appropriate medical training for the Outward Bound instructors working there. They found common ground in a practical and commonsense approach to medicine, and a teaching style and depth of experience well suited to their task. Their early efforts set the stage for Dr. Goth's founding of Wilderness Medical Associates, Inc., and the pair's coauthorship of the first edition of *The Outward Bound Wilderness First-Aid Handbook*. Jeff continues to teach with WMA as a lead instructor, as well as with Outward Bound in both medical and outdoor education roles.